Our daily fix

Sponsored by Alcohol and Drug Foundation, Australia

Our daily fix
Drugs in Australia

Valerie A. Brown · Desmond Manderson
Margaret O'Callaghan · Robyn Thompson

Australian National University Press
A division of Pergamon Press Australia

Australian National University Press is a division of Pergamon Press Australia and a member of the Pergamon Group of Companies.

AUSTRALIA	Pergamon Press (Australia) Pty Ltd, 19a Boundary Street, Rushcutters Bay, N.S.W. 2011, Australia
U.K.	Pergamon Press Ltd, Headington Hill Hall, Oxford OX3 0BW, England
U.S.A.	Pergamon Press Inc., Maxwell House, Fairview Park, Elmsford, N.Y. 10523, U.S.A.
CANADA	Pergamon Press Canada Ltd, Suite 104, 150 Consumer's Road, Willowdale, Ontario M2J IP9, Canada
FEDERAL REPUBLIC OF GERMANY	Pergamon Press GmbH, 6242 Kronberg-Tanus, Hammerweg 6, Postfach 1305, Federal Republic of Germany

First published in Australia 1986 by the Australian National University Press.

Copyright © 1986 Valerie A. Brown, Desmond Manderson, Margaret O'Callaghan, Robyn Thompson

Cover design by Adrian Young

Designed by Ingrid Padina

Typeset in Australia by Rochester Communications Group.
Printed in Australia by Brown Prior Anderson Pty. Ltd.

National Library of Australia Cataloguing in Publication Data

Our Daily Fix

> Bibliography.
> Includes index.
> ISBN 0 08 033044 4.

1. Drug abuse — Australia. 2. Drugs — Australia. I. Brown, Valerie A. II. Title.

362.2'93'0994

All rights reserved. No part of this publication may be reproduced, stored in a retrieval system or transmitted in any form or by any means, electronic, mechanical, photocopying, recording or otherwise without the prior permission of Pergamon Press (Australia) Pty Ltd.

Contents

Preface ix
Foreword xii

PART 1   IDEAS: UNDERSTANDING DRUG USE
1 The world in our heads: totems and taboos 3
2 The social context of drug use 21
3 Drug policy, politics and values 45
4 Effects and extent of drug use 59

PART 2   STRATEGIES: REDUCING DRUG ABUSE
5 Our heads in the world 89
6 Control 97
7 Treatment 116
8 Education 130
9 Social change 141

PART 3   ACTION: BALANCING DRUG USE AND ABUSE
10 Changing the world 165
11 A national campaign against drug abuse 175
    Appendix 1: DA:NA workshop 197
    Appendix 2: Official release from the Special
                 Premiers' Conference on Drugs,
                 Canberra, 2 April 1985 211
12 A national repertoire of action plans 215
13 The heart of the matter 256

Postscript 270
Notes for further reading 273

Bibliography 281
Glossary 297
Index 300

Figures

1	Levels of action on social issues	14
2	One view of marihuana use	19
3	Tic-tac-totem	21
4	Marihuana in the headlines	37
5	Drugs in the headlines	44
6	Heroin in the headlines	103
7	Alcohol in the headlines	160
8	Evaluating the action: a five-sided approach	173
9	Framework for DA:NA	179
10	Drugs in the headlines — again	255
11	A loaded dice?	265
12	Snakes and ladders	266

Tables

1	Royal Commissions, etc.: the 6400 page questions	10
2	Framework for drug issues 1: overview	16
3	Framework for drug issues 2: marihuana	17
4	What counts as a drug problem: a social history	24
5	Patterns of drug use by age	27
6	Politics, values and policy	49
7	Framework for drug issues 3: policy analysis — a binary view	57
8	Most commonly abused chemical substances in Australia in 1985	63
9	Admissions to hospitals with a principal dignosis specifying drug involvement, 1981	73
10	Death rates and drugs, 1974-83	74
11	Drinking patterns among persons aged 25-64 years, Australian State capital cities, 1980 and 1983	75
12	Smoking patterns among persons aged 25-64 years, Australian State capital cities, 1980 and 1983	77
13	Weekly drug use by year 10 students, New South Wales, 1971-83	79

14	Australian Health Surveys, 1977-78 and 1983: persons taking medication in the two days before interview	81
15	Prescriptions form psychopharmaceuticals and total prescriptions under the Pharmaceutical Benefits Scheme, 1974-75 to 1983-84	83
16	Deaths involving drugs reported upon by Sydney Coroner's Court, 1972-80	84
17	Choosing a strategy: collecting the evidence	94
18	Framework for drug issues 4: strategy analysis — responses to heroin use	95
19	Criminal charges associated with specific drugs, 1977-81	113
20	Seizures of selected drugs by Federal agencies, 1977-83	114
21	Framework for drug issues 5: control as policy	115
22	Framework for drug issues 6: treatment as policy	129
23	Framework for drug issues 7: education as policy	139
24	Framework for drug issues 8: prevention as policy	161
25	Ranking of thematic content by press and television, Sydney area, 1984	190
26	Major drug stories of 1984 in Sydney media	191

Cartoons

Pryor: alcohol sponsorship of Melbourne Cup	5
Mitchell: tobacco sponsorship of sport	22
Mitchell: mixed values on alcohol	55
Thaves: prescription of legal drugs	78
Pryor: surveillance as prevention	101
Endean: treatment centres	120
Molnar: marihuana smoking	132
Thaves: effecting social change	148
Thaves: social values	235

Preface

This is a book about reducing the abuse of drugs, through a better understanding of their use. Abuse may be inherited from other parts of the world, or grow out of a homebound tradition; either way, Australians are showing that they have had enough. Political promises, public outcry, and professional criticism are carrying the one message: drug use in Australia has gone beyond the level of our social tolerance. A national campaign against drug abuse was promised by the Prime Minister in November 1984. This was to be designed at a special meeting of the Premiers of the States and Territories in April 1985. Announcement of that meeting stimulated people's awareness of the need to prepare a forceful, realistic brief on their idea of responses to drug use and abuse. One resulting community initiative, sponsored by the Alcohol and Drug Foundation, Australia (ADFA) and the then Capital Territory Health Commission, was 'Drugs in Australia: National Action' (DA:NA), a workshop consisting of forty-four individuals from all States and Territories, selected from the fields of community services, health care, education, law, media and policy analysis. People were invited as individuals with experience of drug use and personal standing in the community, not as representatives of organisations. The DA:NA briefing papers, designed to give participants an overview of current drug use and abuse in Australia, provided the basis of this book; while ADFA has supported publication, the authors take full responsibility for the contents of the book as it now stands.

In the event, the recommendations from the workshop helped set the agenda for the National Campaign meeting, and were reflected in its conclusions. That story is told in Chapter 11. We wish to acknowledge the people who contributed their ideas, their time and their energy to help us bring these papers together. It would not have been possible without the willing help of almost everyone with whom we came in contact during the project. We were continually conscious of the power of a true community initiative. In particular we must thank the following: the organising committee of DA:NA—Professor Ian Webster (Chairman), Dr Valerie Brown, Dr Ken Doust, Dr Les Drew, Dr Jan Fraillon, The Venerable Archdeacon Ian George, Mr Ossie Kleinig, Sir William Refshauge, and Dr Nan Waddy (ADFA President)—and the DA:NA secretariat—Gary Cobcroft, Colleen Crane, Annabell Freeman, Jill Hollands, John Jackson, Robyn Michel, and Colleen Sheen. We had many advisers and consultants—Barbara Allan of ADFA Library, Andy Butlin, Jeannie Ferris, Winifred Garran, George Klein, John Lipsett, Robin McKewan, Lyn Montgomery, and George Van Der Heide—who were exceptionally generous with their respective skills.

Jane Frost was a project officer for DA:NA who worked with us throughout the preparation of the briefing papers and the workshop; her skills as economist, statistician and team mate were invaluable. Members of the Commonwealth Department of Health have given both practical and moral support to this most unbureaucratic of enterprises. Staff of the ACT Health Authority provided the spine of the original workshop, and the Typing Bureau, in particular its chief, Patricia Muir, and Cindy Bell, expertly guided us from briefing papers to book. Ann Neale has carried editing to an art form in her improvement of our manuscript. Members of the Federal Parliament have given us permission to use excerpts from their speeches: Senator Rosemary Crowley, Senator Peter Baume, Ms Ros Kelly and Dr Neal Blewett. Dr Blewett, Commonwealth Minister for Health, supported the workshop throughout. Professor Ian Webster and Dr Earle Hackett have contributed Foreword and Postscript respectively to the book of the workshop. Barbara Allan compiled the index.

We also thank each other. It was demanding of our intellectual and emotional reserves to work so closely together through the briefing papers, workshop design and execution, and the present publication. We are four: Valerie A. Brown, after ten years on the academic staffs of the Human Sciences Program, Australian National University, and Health Studies, Canberra College of Advanced Education, and a Ph.D thesis on methods of relating scientific evidence to social issues, directs the Health Promotion services of the ACT Health Authority; Desmond Manderson has honours in law from the Australian National University with a thesis on the law in relation to social and political change and is completing honours in history; Margaret O'Callaghan taught in primary schools, has been active in community organisations such as the Nursing Mothers Association of Australia, has organised a community service, and has a Bachelor of Applied Science degree in health education from the Canberra College of Advanced Education; Robyn Thompson taught home economics and social psychology at high schools, completed her Bachelor of Education degree at the Canberra College of Advanced Education and tutored there in the sociology of health until becoming project officer (alcohol and drugs) with the Youth and Schools Section of the ACT Health Promotion service. Being different shapes, sizes, sexes, ages, and training, we have had to rub the corners off each other as well as off the material. It has been a rewarding experience.

Finally, we thank the participants of DA:NA whose hard work would refute any cynics who claim there is no sense of community responsibility left. Forty-four people worked unceasingly for three days without tangible reward in order to unite their views on drugs. We dedicate this book to those people and others like them, who care and who act.

Valerie A. Brown
Desmond Manderson
Margaret O'Callaghan
Robyn Thompson

Canberra, July 1985

Foreword

The task

We can't pretend that the task is easy, nor the problem clear. On the one hand, there is public disquiet focused on illicit drug use; yet the use of these drugs cannot be separated from the use of legitimate drugs, mind-altering substances or prescribed medications. Nor can the drug problem be separated from the problems of people.

I recall at a committee meeting in New South Wales the bland item, 'drugs', appeared on the agenda. This was about eight years ago and the person who introduced the item had an axe to grind. As the item was discussed, it was soon evident that the committee had little common ground from which to discuss the issue. The instigator saw the problem as a threat to his kids attending a well-to-do school. He wanted to punish the pushers and users more. With reddened face, he put his case. He pressed the committee to recommend along these lines. The magistrate amongst us could see how counter-productive this would be. Others interpreted the problem from their own experience: through hospital casualty departments, courts, schools, friendships, and so on.

In reading this book you will be asked to test and balance your view against that of others. One of the principal tasks the authors have set themselves is to provide a balanced opinion from informed community spokespersons and specialised research on the nature and extent of drug problems in Australia.

Why now? There are some here who will say that the drug problem is no worse than ten years ago. They will point to evidence that national alcohol consumption has slowed its rise, that deaths due to drugs (especially alcohol and cigarettes) have plateaued, even declined, that special alcohol and drug units have been established in a number of major hospitals, that a number of detoxification units have been established, that a new medical society in this field has been created, and more medical practitioners have specialised in the field.

On the other hand, there is a feeling abroad that the drug problem is undermining our society: threatening the future of young people, escalating drug and organised crime and corrupting our social institutions of law and order and politics. How sensible that perception is, and whether and how we should respond are crucial questions which need to be answered.

Reliefs and fears

Ask any parent of a teenager; visit a Rotary club; speak to schoolteachers; inquire of an inner city GP, and you will learn of their anxiety about their own children, the children of others and the dangers they perceive. Such fears permeate all levels of our society. No one is immune. To be constantly reminded of these risks by the media and public figures provokes a response: it could not be me, my family; they must be mad or criminals; they deserve it; their parents are to blame, and so on. A stereotype is constructed to distance ourselves from the fears of the unknown. The derelict alcoholic becomes the image of alcoholism when, in truth, he/she may be a relative, colleague or friend.

When a group of people are not known, their motivations not understood and they pose a threat, real or imagined, we stereotype them and project negative attributes on to them so as to invalidate their claims and needs. Thus, we deny to ourselves that drug use is intrinsically part of our social relationships, and we ourselves, or people close to us, may be misusing them.

Medically, there are gaps in knowledge as well. What is the natural history of drug use? The question is so fundamental that a special effort is required to find out what actually happens to drug-dependent people. For cigarette smoking we have good information about its contribution to disease, mortality and disabling conditions. But as far as alcohol consumption is concerned, surprisingly little is known about the history of heavy drinkers. Some may move in and out of periods of heavy drinking. Some develop cirrhosis, some brain damage and others are mainly affected by social strife. Why some take these various pathways and not others is very much in the realm of guesswork. For narcotic dependence, the natural remission, death and long-term disability rates are not known. One argument for the registration of narcotic-dependent people is that with such information follow-up studies of the effectiveness of various treatment and rehabilitation programs can be undertaken. It would also allow us to test whether the services provided are matching the demands for them.

Prevention

The first theme of this book is reconciliation of differing views; the second is prevention. The notion that prevention should be part of a public health approach to drug problems is surprisingly recent. And the idea that health concerns extended beyond the conventional stereotype of an 'addict' or an 'alcoholic' to include a spectrum of problems of drug and alcohol use emerged into the public domain in the late 1960s. Up until this time preventive approaches were often opposed by public bodies — especially in the field of alcohol control. The area of prevention offers a significant challenge to propose practical approaches which governments can support and/or implement. Public education is intrinsically part of any preventive approach but it should also be appreciated that control measures of any kind will not be tolerated, let alone work, unless the community is educated about the problem, recognises the need and assents to the introduction of control measures.

It is possible

I have often heard Ted Noffs say that problems offer potentials — potentials for action and alternatives — and that unless you become part of the solution you are part of the problem. If we don't try, who will? Let me restate from the text which follows 'that the greatest obstacle to understanding and responding to behaviour involving drugs is the belief that, because a drug is involved, the behaviour is unique and requires new research, specially trained experts, new and special methods of intervention and treatment'.

What we require are the approaches we apply to the problems of ordinary, non drug-using citizens to be applied ethically, and with justice, to drug problems and to drug users.

The issues we have to grapple with are complex and emotional, and proposals concerning their resolution bring forth strong opinions and biases. This book seeks to chart a way through.

Ian W. Webster
Foundation Professor of Community Medicine
University of New South Wales

Sydney, March 1985

PART 1

IDEAS:
Understanding Drug Use

1
The World in our Heads: Totems and Taboos

Food and drugs

Our daily bread remains symbolic of our very existence, the staff of life, the first thing asked for in a common prayer; the synonym for all food and even for money. We take it orally, daily; we cannot live long without it or its equivalent. Society has legal controls on its content, manufacture and sale.

So what are the differences between drugs and food? We accept that we eat bread and fruit every day and eating them makes us feel good. If a drug is any chemical introduced into the body, and drug abuse is the uncontrolled use of that drug to give personal pleasure, should we say that each of us takes drugs daily? In terms of food we certainly do take it daily, and as consequences of overuse we have obesity, high blood pressure and gall bladder malfunction related to overdoses of sugar, salt and fat.

If we limit the use of the word 'drug' to those chemicals not absorbed for a standard biological purpose, we are still left with a mass of everyday behaviour which falls within the definition. In theory, we use drugs rarely, only when ill or in special need. Yet very few Australians go for two or three days without using a chemical for pleasure, even when we exclude salt and sweeteners. For the young, cola and chocolate drinks; for the older, caffeine, alcohol and nicotine. Advertising leaves us with each of those drugs linked to important central symbols of our culture: the bright young life with a coke drink, the elegant sophisticate with an expensive brand of cigarette. Some are targeted even more closely: banishing potential menstrual pain with the use of aspirin linked to social success for the young woman, and knowing the right drink to order linked with commercial success for the young man.

To arrive at a formal definition of a drug, or a moral standard for what constitutes abuse, is fraught with peril. As a working definition, however, we can agree that any chemical substance introduced into the human body can be called a drug; and for our purposes, we are restricting the word 'drug' to those chemical substances not central to biological function. Abuse, we are assuming, is not a trigger point or a clear line between use and overuse or legal and illegal use, but a phase where the use of the drug for pleasure is bringing emotional, physical or social harm to the individual using it.

In Australia today, we nearly all have our daily bread. Do we all also have our daily fix? If we do, do we need it, and do we abuse it, or are we at risk of abusing it? It is valuable, at this point in our analysis of drug use, to ask the question which starts off so many social gatherings, 'What's yours?' Our choice of drug is so often a reflection of who we are, an emblem of our social group, and an essential element of our day-to-day coping that we never examine our *own* choices. Our fixes can be thundering music and psychedelic lights, the thin air at the top of high mountains, the adrenalin as we parachute through the sky, the power of prayer, or the high from winning a race. The short-term physiological effects are not markedly different from the narcotic, alcoholic or hallucinogenic shift of consciousness. It is with this perspective of drug use as part of the social fabric in which it is found, as part of all our lives, that we look at the nature and extent of drug abuse, and the strategies which attempt to reduce it.

Scenes of confusion

Our Prime Minister wept about his daughter's heroin addiction on national television; this is the same man who was the world record holder for drinking lots of beer quickly. Tourist buses ran to the centre of our largest city to see prepubescent addicts shooting-up night after night; three bus-loads of police sent to the same spot found a mere taxi-full. Our nation's greatest pride is its sporting prowess; its greatest sporting event is a horse race and its greatest sporting triumph a yacht race, and both of them sponsored by brewers.

By mid high school, half of our school students use alcohol weekly. This rate has doubled in the last decade; at the same time consumption by adults has steadied. We have the highest use of painkillers and incidence of kidney disease in the world and tranquilliser prescription is also high. Yet the former has risen by about a third, while the use of tranquillisers has dropped. Statistics which have regularly shown men as the major abusers of alcohol and women of painkillers and tranquillisers are levelling out; yet sex polarisation in employment remains stronger here than in almost any other western country. Clearly, the news is not all bad, but neither is it good enough.

Drugs are part of our lives in individually unique ways. For some—the young and the old, the sick, the unhappy and the dispossessed—they may be chief reason for living. For the rest they are in differing degrees lubricants of rites of passage, the means of celebration in life's triumphs and of comfort in life's despairs. Drugs are crutches, wings, friends, foes, ladders, tunnels. They are the insurance policy for the longest life expectancy humans have ever known, but also the greatest single cause of death and disability in the western world.

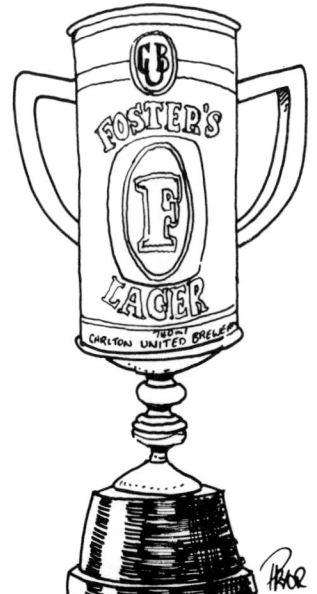

Cartoon by Pryor, reprinted by permission of Pryor of the **Canberra Times,** *from* **Canberra Times,** *2 April 1985*

Totems and taboos

The worlds within the heads of individuals cement communities, and create inconsistencies within a culture, between cultures, and over time. Here and now—as also there and then—the use of drugs as both totem and taboo is woven so deeply into the scripts we carry with us from childhood, and the unspoken rules of how we should behave, that is is extremely difficult to be wise about our own personal decisions on drug taking. More difficult still is the achievement of a balanced view of the drug use of others.

As Levi-Strauss has pointed out, all groups make rules for themselves and enforce the rules by allocating some behaviour to the category of the necessary, a part of the identity of the group, the 'totem' to which all subscribe. These totems, or essential symbols of our society, might be two fully efficient, intelligent, healthy adults and their two fully efficient, intelligent, healthy children. Linked to this is the medication of children, by immunisation, antibiotics and vitamin supplements, so that they realise their full potential in the cult of the individual. The adults in their turn use alcohol as a required social lubricant: 'go on, have another beer mate'; caffeine as an intellectual stimulant; and a range of psychotropic drugs such as sedatives, tranquillisers and antidepressants, to remain at the peak of their performance: 'just take this and you'll be all right'. Legal drugs represent totems of good health, of professional infallibility and of triumph over disease.

These rules and symbols are reinforced even more profoundly by taboos. These are not, as is often misconceived, rules against behaviour. Taboos are a denial that such behaviour could even be considered. Incest and cannibalism are classic examples, behaviours which so threaten the totem family unit that they are regarded as unimaginable. Laws are created to deal with infringements of the totems; but tabooed behaviour is much more treated by society as lawless—denied, ignored and secret.

Thus, the hard statistics that one of the highest occupational risks of drug addiction lies in the health care profession have not been adequately admitted, even to help treat sufferers: such a fact cuts across the totem of drugs of healing dispensed by honoured high priests of medicine, and is taboo. Similarly, the sacred position of alcohol in our society has led to a denial of the enormity of alcohol problems by successive governments, despite report after report and statistic upon statistic. Twenty per cent of hospital admissions are alcohol related, yet to this day most hospitals make no provision for alcohol use or misuse to be listed as the reason for admission. Narcotics viewed today only as taboo have a long history of totemic use. It is not merely a question of other times and other cultures. Such drugs were also totems during the sixties both for anti-war groups and for many soldiers on active service in Vietnam. But their use, well known among the young, is seldom able to be discussed. And heroin addiction remains so severely taboo that neighbouring families have no idea that they have a common problem, and parents deny even to themselves the evidence of their own eyes.

Don't panic

It is this conflict of totem and taboo, the confusion of contradictory images and the clash of inconsistent but sincerely held societal values, that creates much of the problem in dealing with drug use and abuse in Australia today. Aldous Huxley predicted that the Brave New World would use drugs much like cocaine to ease the pain of dying. He has described his amazement that so many of his predictions have already come to pass. Yet we cannot decide the future we want while the present remains an undeciphered code. Faced with confusion and paradox, it would be easy to panic. Parents care about their children, children care about their future, and the community cares about its values and beliefs.

Don't panic. The basic questions remain vital and answerable. We can examine the who, what, where, when and why of drug taking. Who are the drug takers? What ages, groups, stereotypes, sexes or occupations show what patterns of drug use and abuse with what drug and under what conditions? What drugs are consumed in Australia today, for what purposes, and with what benefits to whom?

Where do drugs come from and where do they go? Are the subgroups in society which show divergent patterns of drug use—like the Cedar Bay bush dwellers expelled from their tropical retreat by Queensland police in 1978—unacceptable to us? Should the different attitudes to drugs within different groups and cultures affect our response to such groups or to the drugs?

When drugs are taken is a crucial element of understanding. Weil in *The natural mind* describes the subjective and personal nature of the effects on the human body of an interfering chemical substance. The time of life, the time of day, the physical and social environment and, perhaps most powerfully of all, the contemporary social view of a particular drug can affect its physiological effect on an individual. People's reaction to nicotine, and the strength of its addictive hold, is dependent on these factors, as is people's response to and tolerance of chemotherapy in the treatment of cancer. A historical context, too, will determine the conditions under which a drug is taken and social reaction to it. The gin mills of Hogarth and 'gin a penny' of the eighteenth century contrast with the planter's gin of the colonial era and the faintly decadent aura of gin-and-tonic today.

Key to deciphering: practical knowledge

Throughout this book, an attempt is made to deal with these basic questions. The most important steps in resisting the rising tide of panic and seeking the key to the cipher are to become informed in a balanced way on drug issues, and to be aware of the moral conflict and values involved. The world in the head and the world of things can be charted. There are studies, observations, and initiatives which allow a balanced view of drug issues, and the evidence to arrive at a middle ground on which decisions can be made.

Yet what is dramatically clear about the many reports and commissions that have been conducted in recent years is the similarity of so many of their findings (see Table 1). The commissions were divided on the following points: methadone maintenance, penalties for the use and possession of cannabis, compulsory treatment. There was total or significant agreement on: co-ordination of agencies, centralised intelligence, need for more and co-ordinated research and statistics, a multi-faceted approach to attainable goals, no significant increase in police powers or stricter laws except phone interception, pre-sentence assessment and diversion, past exaggeration of cannabis risks, and the importance of alcohol as a major drug abuse problem. Most other issues covered by the commissions received similar comments in more than one report and no dissent in the others.

Perhaps the similarity of findings is indicative of an overeagerness to conduct inquiries rather than act. It is clear at least that the knowledge of experts has not filtered down to the community. Yet this step is vital.

It is fair to say that there has been much talk and little action. If commissioners are agreed on most things, and if the things about which they disagree are so well defined, why has there been so little positive effect? It is not a failure of knowledge alone, but of communication, for the five interrelated elements of drug behaviour (though often treated in isolation) are easily identified:

(a) the drug—the intruding chemical
(b) the drug user—patient, addict, client, spouse, child, person
(c) the drug supplier—multinational drug company, Mafia ring, medical practitioner, family member, corner store
(d) the drug-taking activity—Friday night pub crawl, examination swot, coffee break, solitary injection, surgery visit, intensive care ward
(e) social symbolism of the drug—totem or taboo.

The first three approaches are the more common ways to understanding drugs and the pharmacology and physiological effects of most drugs are well understood. Summary tables of drugs and their effects are provided in Chapter 4, 'Effects and extent of drug use'. The long search for a description of the 'typical' drug user has ended in a draw, however. Demographic profiles of who is prone to use what drugs are also provided, in Chapter 2; but while predisposing agents for drug use have been identified to include an absent or alcoholic parent or other childhood traumas, myths of a stereotypical drug-addicted personality, group or environment have been exploded. It is generally accepted that drug behaviour relates to the individual social purposes of the user, as expanded on in Chapter 2, 'The social context of drug use'. It is essentially a moral judgment within society's social symbolism whether such behaviour is considered to be use or abuse of the chemical substance. The inconsistency of this symbolism and morality within a culture and between cultures and over time is also dealt with in Chapter 2. Chapter 3, 'Drug policy, politics and values' explores how the differing moral standpoints within a society affect views on how to deal with basic and vital questions of drug use, such as the control of the individual and the aims and

Table 1
Royal Commissions, etc. : the 6400 page questions

RECOMMENDATION	S.S.C.	BAUME	WOODWARD	WILLIAMS	SACKVILLE	STEWART	OTHER
POLICY AND PRIORITY							
Psycho-social approach	●●	●					●●● Le Dain
Treatment-user; control traffic	●●	●					●●● Le Dain
Distinguish narcotics from cannabis			●	●			● Shafer
Support for international supply efforts	All reports: Esp. in Woodward, Sackville and Le Dain						
Need for attainable goals			●	●			● Le Dain
Increased resources for supply controls							
Importance of alcohol	Emphasised as the most serious problem in all reports					●	
STRATEGIES AND TACTICS							
Lower excise for LA beer	●	●●●●					● HRC
Advertising ban on tobacco and alcohol							
No grants to organ. with tobacco/alcohol funding							
Mechanical devices for drink drivers							● HRC
Therapeutic communities favoured							
Methadone programs			●	O●●●●	●		● Le Dain
Continue heroin ban unless analgesic advantage				●●	●●●		● Le Dain
Community involvement	●						
Use mainly of voluntary organisations	●			●			● Le Dain
Control of ads. to medical profession							
Cannabis options							
No change pending research					●		
Destroy convictions							
Decriminalisation		●●	●●				●● Oregon.Calif
Partial legislation							●● Le Dain

THE WORLD IN OUR HEADS: TOTEMS AND TABOOS

Proposition							Source
Drug education							
Need to target groups				•			Le Dain
Need for a broad health education in schools			•	•		• •	Le Dain
Drug training for medical professionals							
PROCEDURES							
Assessment and diversion (Baume recommends this for cannabis, but others do not)			• • •			•	Le Dain
No mandatory sentences			• • •	• •			
No compulsory interrogation				○			
Compulsory treatment outside criminal law				•		•	Le Dain
No general warrants			• • •				
Interception in trafficking on judicial warrant				•			
Limited use of intrusive body searches						•	Lusher
Guarding against police corruption							
No change in bail laws							
National Strategy on Drug Abuse:							
Use of the phrase			• •	• • • • •	•	• •	Moffitt
Forces and agencies co-ordination					•	• •	Moffitt / Hope
Intelligence and information co-ordination			• •				
Legal consolidation	• •		• • ○			•	HRC
Research and statistics, database and co-ord.							HRC / Le Dain
Co-ordinated research into cannabis and driving	•						
National Crimes Commission	• •						

KEY

The report—
● agreed with this proposition
○ disagreed with this proposition
🐢 unsure of this proposition

Sources for this table are in the Bibliography. HRC is Australia, House of Representatives Standing Committee on Road Safety; SSC is Australia, Senate Select Commission of Drug Trafficking and Drug Abuse.

priorities of a drug abuse campaign. These broad questions are vital in any rational and coherent approach to drugs.

The topic of the supply of drugs is a matter for economists, criminologists and sociologists. Although touched upon in Chapters 6 and 7, 'Control' and 'Treatment', this aspect is not explored in depth. We are more concerned with extending our understanding of drug use and in exploring the social conditions under which drug use can be of maximum benefit and its misuse under maximum control. Chapters 6 and 7, and Chapters 8 and 9, 'Education' and 'Social change', contain a review and an evaluation of strategies currently available to prevent misuse.

Key to deciphering: a will to act

The knowledge for synthesis of actions and ideals is available. So is the will. Even in a country as factionalised as Australia, there is a counterbalancing concern for the national, community and personal good. An election promise by that same tearful Prime Minister was met by a wave of community-initiated consultation. Five hundred and seven submissions were produced in six weeks, accompanied by grass roots conferences all over the country, official consultations with the States and Territories and a national drug workshop with the goal of co-ordinating community priorities. The story of how forty-four people from all States of Australia, from law, medicine, education, policy analysis and the media, and from a range of backgrounds, ages and experience, attacked the questions of drug abuse is related in Chapter 11, 'A national campaign against drug abuse', where we examine the difficulties and values of such a community enterprise.

For this same national drug workshop, project officers summarised the mass of material on drug use published as special reports, popular works and academic treatises. Those summaries are woven into the present book. For those who wish to consult the sources, these are listed in the Bibliography and the short annotated reading list. Details of commonly abused drugs can be found in Figure 13.

The will to achieve some progress and understanding on drug issues can also be seen in the many and varied programs in which the community is involved. A range of these is considered in Chapter 12, 'A national repertoire of action plans'. These show that change and balance are possible, but they also indicate that the workings of programs must continually be evaluated against the goals to which they aspire.

Framework for analysis

Unless we can devise frameworks by which we can analyse the many elements of the drug problems, identified above, we will remain in the same state of mental and emotional chaos. There are notable contributors to this task, on whose work we can draw. Helen Nowlis of USA has given insights into the fixed perspectives on drug use in western culture, and the options for action; she identifies the four strategies by which we attempt to reduce abuse at present and the split between seeing drug use as a problem and as a part of society. Les Drew has examined the value priorities in the Australian community. Peter Baume and Robin Room have studied Australian drug use patterns and identified this nation as an intoxicated society.

Part of the framework that we will use has already been outlined. In this book we recognise that any effective understanding of drugs, proceeding to action, must carefully co-ordinate three levels. Thus:

POLICY   Health is an inalienable human right; cigarette smoking is a proven health hazard and therefore to be discouraged.
Note: a statement of principle.

STRATEGY   Concentrate on discouraging smoking in public places.
Note: a statement which links values and practice.

ACTIONS   Conduct health education campaigns in the work place; legislate to stop smoking in lifts and public transport; provide support for smokers to stop.
Note: a statement of practice.

These levels alone are not enough. All three need to be considered in relation to a fourth, often ignored, but equally vital: the social context in which they are set. It is this social context which determines what can realistically be done and achieved. So we can add a fourth level:

SOCIAL CONTEXT Society recognises the personal freedom to smoke but does not accept a right to intrude on the freedom of others; modern society is stressful, and social supports such as stable families and secure employment are decreasing. *Note: a statement of controls, attitudes and conflicting values.*

Chapter 2 deals with *social context*, Chapter 3 with *policy*, Chapter 4 with *statistics* of drug use (the basic ideas); Chapters 6–9 the various aspects of current *strategies for reducing drug abuse*; and Chapters 10–12 the details of effective *actions* available. Many programs do exist which embody strategies which have no policy basis, and similarly policies often ignore the social context in which they have to operate. The result of omitting any of these considerations is obviously not ideal, since these levels are not independent of one another. Interrelationships are suggested in Figure 1.

Policy and social context are interdependent and so need to be both compatible and *consistent*. Which strategies are successful in implementing a policy will also depend on their *fit* with social context. Each strategy becomes real only when put into *practical*

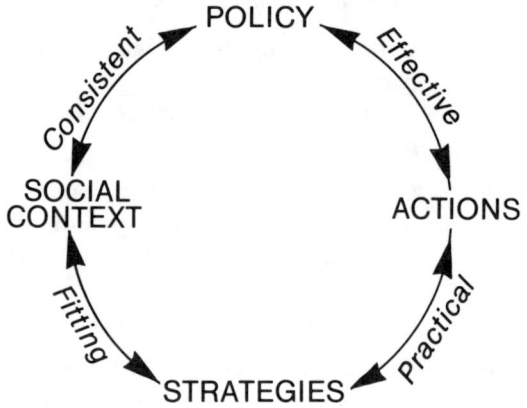

Figure 1   Levels of action on social issues

action. And in the final analysis, the success of a policy will be determined by the long-term *effectiveness* of action taken.

As well as considering all the spokes in the action wheel of Figure 1, it is necessary to make use of all the avenues of response available to deal with a drug problem, that is, all the usual *avenues of response* of legal control, treatment, education and social change. For example:

Control	Limit times at which alcohol can be sold	
Treatment	Provide detoxification units	
Education	Join Alcoholics Anonymous	⎤
		⎥ *Prevention*
Social Change	Community acceptance of light alcohol (LA) beer	⎦

These areas are dealt with, notably in the section on strategies, Chapters 6, 7, 8 and 9, since programs at present tend to run along this division. Tradition puts these four areas into the laps of law, medicine, education and government: lawyer, doctor, indian, chief. This, however, narrows the range of effective actions. For any one issue we need to consider all the levels of action, and all the avenues of approach and response.

The framework in Table 2 can be used in many ways to help clarify the complex issues involved in drug problems; for example, see Table 3.
The use of this analysis is explained further with particular emphasis on policy in Chapter 3. Here it is valuable to note how such an analysis helps explain the relationship of the various factors in the drug debate. It can be seen, for example, that the social context, a time of social change, has stopped the creation of a satisfactory policy; and that the effect of the absence of policy on treatment is a lack of specific response to cannabis use, in strategy and action. Only the secondary consequences of harm (such as a car accident involving drug-affected drivers) are dealt with. A clear and coherent framework is vital because of the sheer weight and gravity of questions relating to drug use. Ponder on these fundamental questions posed by the Organising Committee of a national drug workshop, Drugs in Australia : National Action (DA:NA).

Table 2
Framework for drug issues 1 : overview

	AVENUES OF RESPONSE			
	Control	Treatment	Education	Social change
Policy				
Social context				
Strategy				
Action				

Table 3
Framework for drug issues 2: marijuana

	Avenues of approach			
	Control	Treatment	Education	Social change
Policy	Preferred response: to protect citizens.	None. Users do not exist.	Early warning: do not start.	Controversy—no policy.
Social context	Desire of law abiders to be protected from deviants.	Users don't want treatment; society doesn't want to know.	School is a tool for social conformity.	Loggerheads—some for, some against.
Strategy	Heavy trafficking penalties.	Only secondary consequences of use treated.	Anti-marijuana campaigns.	Opposing campaigns.
Action	Arrest sellers, fine users.	No direct action.	Films and course material.	Lobbies and demonstrations.

Underlying issue
What kind of society do we want in Australia, especially in relation to drug use and abuse?

More particular questions
1. Is there a serious gap between policy makers and our community on the following issues:
   (a) decriminalisation of personal use of cannabis?
   (b) criminalisation of the use of certain drugs?
   (c) rehabilitation of offenders?
   (d) should there be an authorised supply of drugs of addiction, e.g. methadone or heroin?
2. Are there aspects in our legal, economic, political, and education systems preventing the resolution of the problem?
3. What are the advantages of formalised national policies on licit and illicit drugs of addiction? What is required to define and establish such national policies and strategies?
4. Is there enough information about programs to determine those that are effective and the existing gaps? How can we achieve a co-ordinated and complete drug intelligence information base in order to determine effective measures and existing gaps?
5. Can the lessons learnt from our approach to tobacco and alcohol be applied to illicit drugs? How can we learn from other countries?
6. Can we demystify the community beliefs about and attitudes to the use of illicit drugs?
7. How can the community be involved and empowered in the resolution of drug and related problems?
8. What are some of the practical preventive strategies which can be implemented now?
9. How can a balance be achieved between individual rights and public interests?
10. Are special measures required for Aboriginal and other groups?

11. How can the media assist in resolving these problems?
12. Are there community alternatives to the non-therapeutic use of drugs?

To answer questions so fundamental to our society, a rational and effective approach to drug problems must deal with three aspects.

The first, the moral and theoretical aspects of drug issues, are the questions to be asked in understanding the social context of drug use and the formulation of policy. This is dealt with in Part 1, 'Ideas'. Ideas are a whole world—a world in our heads. Ideas are based on fact; but facts are ideas, too. Both are needed for forming a successful policy on drug use.

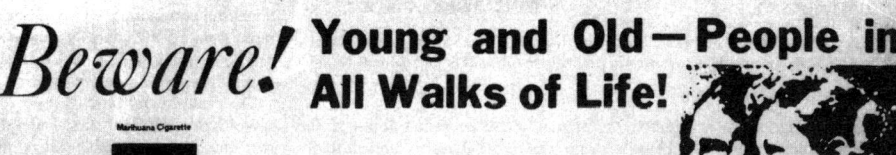
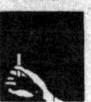

Figure 2   One view of marijuana use

The third aspect covers plans for the effective action required to implement the steps decided by policy. This is dealt with in Part 3, 'Action'—but before we can try and change the world, we must interpret the way the world is, and take the middle step, the bridge of decision making between ideas and action. The nature and extent of the drug problem, and of the various strategies available to implement policy, must be related to the ideas of the individual and the social values of the community. The result is a better understanding of contemporary drug issues, and an ability, therefore, to see better how to take action to reduce abuse. This middle step of translation gives us the Strategies dealt with in Part 2.

While these issues must, of course, be considered by governments, health care and legal professionals and educators, in this book we also aim to encourage personal and community empowerment and access to information, to use analysis as a step towards synthesis, discussion of theories as a step towards effective practice, and to collate specialist opinions as a step along the road to your own understanding.

2
The Social Context Of Drug Use

Playing the game

The social context of drugs is often ignored. Yet the values of a society, the central attitudes which prescribe and proscribe, are central to an understanding of the causes of and responses to drug-taking behaviour. Even those who do consider such questions may approach the matter too superficially: society regards legal drugs almost exclusively as totems, illegal drugs as taboo, and has not yet, maybe, properly decided on cannabis. Is it not then like some crazy game of tic-tac-toe in which society's insistence on these perspectives means that only 'noughts' can win? (See Figure 3.)

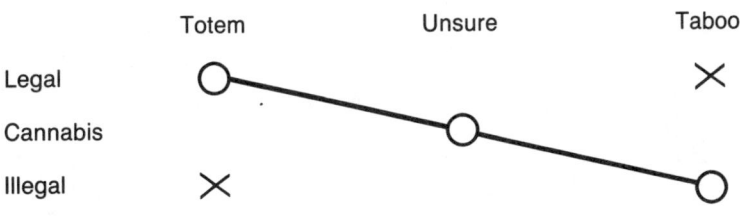

Figure 3   Tic-tac-totem

Yet the situation is a great deal more complex. Alcohol is in Australia today strongly totemised, while heroin is taboo. For each individual drug we may find varying behaviours are approved and disapproved. To further complicate matters, drug use and its social symbolism vary depending on the age of user, the culture of use, and the historical time. A drug which is totem in one culture, such as coca chewing in the Andes, is taboo in another. Within a culture, too, different subgroups have different social values: cocaine sniffing was clearly a totem—or essential symbol—of various wealthy, fashionable, upwardly-mobile circles in Hollywood and New York, yet in much of the rest of society its use was and is condemned not only because it is a 'hard drug' but because of the associated expense and elitism. Understanding the conjunction of totem and taboo, two sides of the same sculpturing of a society, is a vital part of understanding the social context in which drug use and abuse occur.

In this chapter the social basis of drug problems is discussed in some detail. It is also important to note the exacerbation of drug misuse by the very entrenchment of drug use. The place of beer in Australian society, and the place of alcohol and tobacco sponsorship in Australian sport, so entrench drug use as a natural part of what it means to be a Good Australian that the line between what is 'acceptable' and 'unacceptable' in drug use is hopelessly blurred. Said the son of Fred Nile, Festival of Light campaigner:

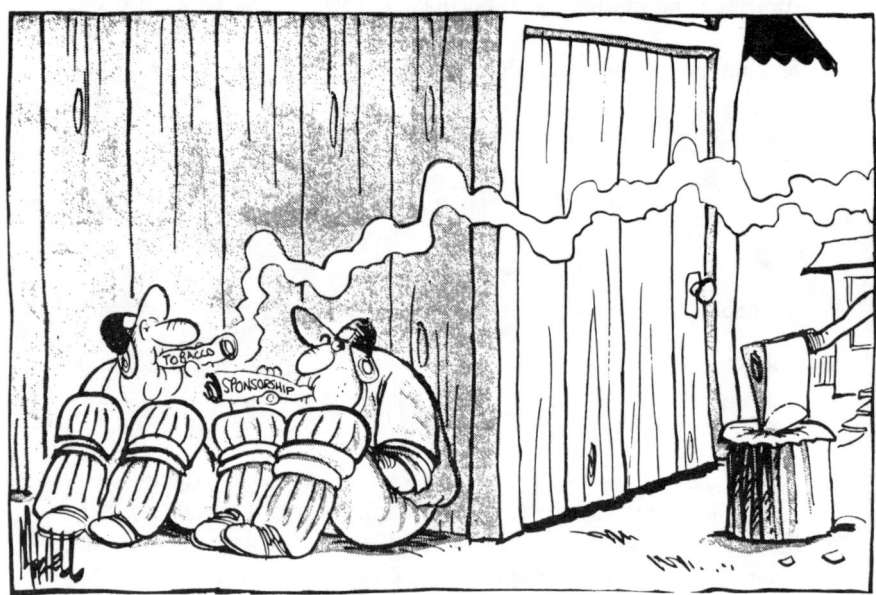

Cartoon by Mitchell, reprinted by permission of the artist, from ***Australian****, 12 October 1984*

'I've never tried marijuana. Never had the urge to. I'm a beer drinker.'

Drug use changes over time

Drug use and social attitudes are not static. What is totemised in one society, at one time, is taboo elsewhere. This much is clear from Table 4. Awareness of the effect that transient values have on what constitutes acceptable and unacceptable drug behaviour is vital to an understanding of contemporary drug problems.

How then does society cope with drug *abuse* when the role of drugs differs so much from culture to culture?

It has been fashionable in Europe to see drug abuse as a product of alienation from mainstream society. It was a popular idea that the drug abuser was an isolate, as for example Sherlock Holmes, Timothy Leary, Thomas De Quincey, Samuel Taylor Coleridge or Sigmund Freud. Considerable social evidence indicates that the isolated drug user was not the norm. 'Alienation' when applied to drug abuse might be better used in reference to the alienation of the practice from other societal practices. This would make the behaviour special but not abnormal.

Thus, drug use in small-scale traditional societies has been well integrated into medicinal, religious, social, recreational or initiation roles. There are exceptions, but for the most part traditional use is 'normal' within that cultural context. For example, as illustrated in Table 4, cannabis smoking among Jamaican workers, chewing coca leaves among Andean Indians, pitcheri use by Aborigines, Datura use by Navajo Indians.

Drugs in either traditional or changing social settings make similar contributions to the lives of individuals and groups within those settings. Drugs have religious and social meanings, functional meanings, medical significance and economic benefits. It is when the clash of drugs as both totem and taboo results in inconsistencies that drugs and drug-taking behaviour are recognised as leading to problems. We also have the puzzling phenomenon that some drug users (like heroin addicts) become visible as such, while others (like lonely mothers taking tranquillisers) are less socially visible. The clash of totem and taboo often leads to a refusal to acknowledge that Australians *do* have a daily fix—but Table 5 shows the continuing patterns of drug use which predominate throughout the life cycle.

Table 4
What counts as a drug problem: a social history

Era	What is happening	Social attitudes to drug use
2000 B.C. -1000 A.D.	COCA chewing in Peru. CANNABIS in India and Iran. OPIUM use in Middle East. TOBACCO smoking in Nth. America. BETELNUT chewing in PNG. DRUNKENNESS in Rome. KHAT chewing in Yemen.	**MYSTIC RITES** Religious and cultural approval and significance. Drug use is integrated into the social fabric.
500 B.C. -500 A.D.	**ALCOHOL** INDIA — Hinduism banned high caste alcohol consumption. CONFUCIANISM — frowned on drinking. **Gender differences** INDIA and ROME — Women not permitted to drink alcohol.	**CLEANSING THE TEMPLE** Development of religious philosophies which frowned upon alcohol.
1600	**TOBACCO** James I considered it to be disgusting. Banned in Turkey because of fires in Constantinople. Users threatened with imprisonment in China. Forbidden in Russia because of bad breath.	**GIN A PENNY** Sanctions to protect hygiene and public safety of autocrats. Drug use in private an acceptable lifestyle. Alcoholism rampant among the poor.

THE SOCIAL CONTEXT OF DRUG USE 25

1800	**OPIUM** Largely accepted in Europe and USA. Samuel Coleridge, Sherlock Homes and Dr William Halsted — famous opium addicts.	**ECCENTRICITY RULES** Some moral sanctions (e.g. 'You sinners') but no legal sanctions.
1890	**OPIUM** Growing trend to prohibition.	**FILTHY FOREIGN HABITS** Large-scale racism directed to minority and immigrant drug habits. Effect in US was — criminals out of addicts largely created by over-medication in Civil War. Self-fulfilling prophesy of 'dope fiends'.
1919-60	**ALCOHOL** Prohibition 1919-33. **MARIJUANA** — *'THE FORBIDDEN FRUIT'* In the wake of anti-narcotic suppression marijuana went along for the ride.	**SPEAKEASY CRIMINALS** The criminalisation of marijuana based on ignorance. Racist overtones (as with opium). Drug use perceived to be a lower class activity; harsh sanctions approved.
1960	**MARIJUANA** — *'THE TREE OF KNOWLEDGE'* Dramatic increase in the use of L.S.D. and marijuana amongst the middle class. **HEROIN** — No 'big deals'. But drug use generally was becoming more diversified: varying use of amphetamines, barbiturates.	**AGE OF AQUARIUS** Social protest. Drug use a response to the 'social climate' — Hippy era and Vietnam war. Drug penalties became a public issue because it's happening to 'us' and not just 'them'. Heroin was illegal in Australia from 1956 but was not a large problem.

Table 4 (continued)

1970-80	**HEROIN** — Increased use. Continuing trend towards poly drug use.	**THE JUNKIE** Social sign of: Response to political and social disillusionment? Existence of a 'pluralistic society'. Much role conflict. EARLY 1970s — Individual seen to be 'diseased' (Public Health Model). Emphasis on naive drug education policies (information and 'cures', e.g. methadone). LATE 1970s — Individual seen as a 'sociopath'. Emphasis therefore on stricter penalties and control (e.g. methadone). EARLY 1980s — Individual seen as a victim of social oppression. Emphasis therefore on 'patronising treatment' (e.g. methadone).
1985 and beyond	COCA chewing in Peru. CANNABIS in India and Iran. OPIUM use in Middle East. TOBACCO smoking in Nth. America. BETELNUT chewing in PNG. DRUNKENNESS in Rome KHAT chewing in Yemen.	**THE PROBLEM THAT WON'T GO AWAY** Social signposts: (a) intolerance and stricter controls or (b) ignoring the problem and neither treating nor controlling or (c) recognition of wider social influence on drug use.

US trends — Australia followed

Table 5
Patterns of drug use by age

	In utero	Infant 0–5	Child 5–12	Adolesc. 12–20	Young adults 20–35	Middle life 35–50	Middle aged 50–65	Older people 65+
	Virtually all drugs affect unborn foetus	·Minor tranquillisers ·Sweeteners	·Sweeteners ·Caffeine (in soft drinks)	Glues Volatile substances ·Cannabis ·Tobacco ·Alcohol ·Caffeine Minor tranquillisers Stimulants Narcotics Polydrug use Alcohol and minor tranquillisers (mixed) Amyl nitrate Compound analgesics	Narcotics ·Cannabis ·Alcohol ·Caffeine ·Tobacco Minor tranquillisers ·Cocaine Stimulants ·Sweeteners Polydrug use Alcohol and minor tranquillisers (mixed)	·Alcohol ·Caffeine ·Tobacco ·Sweeteners Cocaine Minor tranquillisers Compound analgesics Alcohol and minor tranquillisers (mixed)	·Alcohol Minor tranquillisers ·Tobacco ·Caffeine Symptomatic prescribed drugs	·Alcohol ·Tobacco ·Caffeine ·Sweeteners Symptomatic prescribed drugs
Crisis points during the life cycle	TRUST VS MISTRUST	AUTONOMY VS DOUBT	INITIATIVE VS GUILT	INDUSTRY VS INFERIORITY	IDENTITY VS IDENTITY CONFUSION	INTIMACY VS ISOLATION	GENERATIVITY VS STAGNATION	INTEGRITY VS DESPAIR

· = Major drug.
Source: Based on clinical observations at Bourke St. Drug Advisory Centre, Sydney. The crisis points are based on Erikson (1968), pp. 91-135.

Consider the following questions:
1. Which drugs continue through the life cycle?
2. What functions do they perform?
3. What nutrition-supporting function do these drugs have?
4. What factors make these drugs 'attractive' at certain stages of life?

If we all 'do it' (as the above information reveals) why are there so many cultural inconsistencies which render some drugs sacred cows and others fair game for attack?

Rainbow coloured glasses

Jaffe attempts to sort out the dilemma:

> We cannot draw any precise line between 'appropriate' drug use and drug abuse. There is a large grey area open to different interpretations according to the social and cultural background of the interpreter. Different points of view are formulated within a particular cultural setting and may assign quite different meanings to the behaviour in question (page 105).

Moreover, not only are viewpoints dependent on the culture in which they develop, but they can vary dramatically between individuals in that society too.

Thus drugs cause much anxiety and ambivalence and share a history of negative and positive moral evaluation in our society. According to Whyte, because of this ambivalence we come into the area of conflict where personal choice clashes with public values; where our attitudes toward drug taking may not be in accordance with the community's idea of health; where individuals do not wish to change their behaviour, yet the community demands change. And finally, where individual or public ideas of what constitutes a problem do not accord with the law. Whyte reminds us that we all possess a pocket full of different coloured spectacles which we may use to look at others who engage in controversial activities.

Using black tinted spectacles we may see a moral/legal problem and regard the user as ignorant, misguided and wicked and in need of moral education and perhaps punishment. With red tinted specs we adopt a disease or public health stance and see the user as sick, afflicted, diseased and to be treated as a medical problem. Through green spectacles, it is seen as a matter of personal responsibility.

You are free to choose and act as you wish, but on the basis of adequate awareness and education, having a clear appreciation of personal values, and the ability to make decisions and act 'appropriately'. Blue spectacles show it in a socio-cultural light. What can you expect in such a society? There will be casualties, and what the situation calls for is political action, community development and social engineering rather than any focus on the individual.

Table 4 is useful here as a chronology of drug-taking activities. The first step is to recognise that other moral values do exist, and have some validity. The figure highlights the fact that fixed visions can dominate whole eras. It shows the governing images which emerge in specific material and ideological contexts and it shows that governing images of substance use differ from one society to another, and also shift over time. The consequent treatment modalities finally result in 'appropriate' political, economic and gate-keeping mechanisms to deal with the anomalous drug behaviour, and help to shape the society itself.

The fix we're in

Blinkered visions and the tyranny of history are but two of the many ways of shaping our social structure. There are also structural elements which determine the rate and type of drug use. The community to which one belongs will have vested interests, lobby groups, firm opinions about what is education and sources of power and control. Even the ways we are allowed to fix the fix are circumscribed.

Vested interest

The entrenchment and permeation of drugs in Australia are described by Robin Room in *An intoxicated society? Alcohol issues then and now in Australia*. Room puts the spotlight on the power of the legal drug, alcohol, and accuses the alcoholic beverage industry of allying with opinion leaders and the media and identifying themselves with and tying their fortunes to positive features of Australian life and culture. The alcohol industry, even more so than the tobacco industry, has been assigned the same status as our top sporting heroes.

This vested interest in our community which seeks maintenance of the status quo for social or financial reasons can inhibit positive change. The alcohol and tobacco industries are involved; so are the drug companies, pushers, addicts, pharmacists, politicians, media, advertising, professional people, police and law enforcement agencies, and the government with its tobacco subsidies and excise revenue.

Lack of trust
Mistrust is another entrenchment agent and an impediment which inhibits any resolution of drug problems. Within and between agencies, institutions and individuals there is a lack of trust and co-operation at all levels. Inter-department rivalries abound, people withhold information. As a result there is undue loss of life and morbidity, the facilitation of bitterness, despair and powerlessness in both clients and care workers, breakdown in effectiveness, tendency for empire building, pervasive insecurity about the maintenance and continuity of programs and funding failures which often lead to 'quick fix' programs.

The professionals in general mistrust the media; the media in turn grasp at the sensational, the here and now and the trivial in the absence of co-operative policies. The politician is left poorly, ambiguously and irrationally informed.

Fear and ignorance
Widespread fear and ignorance concerning drugs in our society lead to a range of actions which are self-fulfilling and promote further ignorance. These include 'them' and 'us' attitudes, stereotyping, polarisation, denial, stigmatisation, role assumptions and coercion into roles, imposition of values, imposition of a supposed 'norm' as distinct from valuing and respecting individual differences, and a bias towards the formation of vulnerable groups in defence.

Dependence
Dependence (the process of addiction) is a far wider issue than the end result, of which active drug taking is only one form. Other responses include various unconstructive approaches to living which do not address living skills and strengths coming from the

individual as an active participant in society. We are all part of the process of dependence.

The use and abuse of drugs within society are therefore attempts by some to find a solution to this broader problem. The nature of the problem is one of dependence; our expectations that life's problems/failures can be solved by external forces rather than by individual resources. Some people therefore become dependent upon drugs whereas others maintain different (perhaps more acceptable) dependences. Irrespective of the solution sought, there is an underlying propensity to be dependent, with a significant proportion of the population turning towards drug dependence. 'Drugs' used as the mechanism to fulfil this potential dependence include aspirin, alcohol, tobacco, TV, as well as illicit drugs.

Dependence leads to deprivation of civil rights, as visibly drug-dependent people are devalued by society (as represented by professionals, law enforcement agencies, health providers), and are subject to inconsistencies in the provision of services. Discriminatory attitudes lead in turn to authoritarian solutions which further erode independence.

Drug problems are people problems

Drug problems are rarely caused simply by drug use. More often, drugs are a mainspring of action and many social problems are manifested in drug problems. Too often the focus is on the drug or the user and the problems of the consequences of substance use. The community at times becomes so befuddled by the stereotype that the identity of the person taking the drugs and the problems of origin of the abuse are often ignored. But clearly, drug problems are people problems. We can roughly describe the characteristics of some groups at particularly high risk of drug abuse. But this information is of no value for understanding the issues if it is read as descriptions of stereotypes. Any one of us could, under some conditions, have fallen into one of the categories (drawn from Stanton, and Wesson and Smith).

This list is by no means exhaustive. Other likely groups of drug users include single mothers, isolated elderly people, sports people, students, single fathers, prostitutes, homeless young men and women.

Narcotics Users

Some group characteristics
age range from as young as 13-40+
legal problems
physical health problems

Social context
media sensationalised
sub-culture of fashionable heroin abuse
widespread legal addiction

Young Unemployed

Some group characteristics
social isolation/low self-esteem
poor housing, poor prospects, poor nutrition
at risk of drug involvement both for euphoria and financial gain
widespread use of alcohol

Social context
occupation as a measure of self-esteem
community verbally concerned but fragmented

Homeless Children

Some group characteristics
need for peer groups and parental support
physical health poor
self-esteem low—sense of not belonging
attraction of 'ghetto'—inner city as visible gathering point
experimentation with whole range of drugs, especially among males
sexual experimentation
attraction to prostitution
drug sales as a source of income, and provision of a sense of occupation and lifestyle

Social context
community verbally concerned but fragmented
media sensationalised
some parental cases of sexual and physical abuse

Families of drug users

Some group characteristics
confused/ambivalent about their appropriate role
tendency to form alliances within the family
tendency to have family history of drug use
guilt, shame, feelings of obligation
frustration, anger and confusion leading to hopelessness, marital breakdown, etc.

Social context
widespread acceptance that child care is the domain of mothers
isolation of family as economic unit
widespread acceptance of peer alcoholism among males
parents poorly resourced

Ethnic Drug Users
(especially young adult males—Maltese, Lebanese, Yugoslav, Greek, Italian, Turkish, etc.)

Some group characteristics
incomplete or poor understanding of cultural mechanisms including language, social practices, educational options, etc.
close-knit involvement with family and ethnic community in ghetto type situation
incentive of drug sales as source of economic gain, thereby increasing self-esteem.

Social context
widespread unemployment
few job opportunities without qualifications
'competitiveness' as a social barrier in wider society (you are taking 'our' jobs)
many have parents in another country where civil war prohibits contact; making money becomes an urgency

Aboriginal Drug Users

Some group characteristics
widespread use of alcohol; also some use of solvents
detribalised, but communal social practices in towns/cities
values profoundly at odds with other urban lifestyles
welfare payments, main source of income

Social context
uninterest/disapproval from rest of society
active segregation
some contempt for the Aboriginal person because 'they can't hold their liquor'

Politicians also care

At a time of national concern about drugs and their problems, it is not surprising to find many politicians making statements on the issues involved. The papers presented to DA:NA by four members of the Australian Federal Parliament, from both upper and lower houses, Labor and Liberal Parties, are a useful guide to political thinking at that time.

These four speeches, coming as they do from a present and a past Minister for Health, from State and local representatives and from in and out of government, show only minor differences of emphasis. Remarkable is their agreement on the major issues, at a time when the same parties are sharply divided over a range of other issues, such as the use of nuclear power, Aboriginal land rights and private versus public education.

The central points made in each of the four speeches were also reflected in the recommendations of the participants at the end of the workshop. Excerpts from the politicians' speeches are included below and the full recommendations from the workshop are included in Chapter 11. Taking these together it seems fair to conclude that the social context of drug use in Australia is as follows:

(a) our daily fixes of alcohol, aspirin and nicotine have by far the most worrying consequences
(b) we have made some headway with lowering abuse of legal drugs, but have not even started on reducing the criminalisation of our society associated with the sharp increase in the use of illegal drugs
(c) control of supply and use of drugs is necessary, but we would be naive if we considered that control measures alone are solutions to the problem
(d) drug abuse is a community problem, not a foreign import, and it cannot be solved without the support of community agencies and active community intervention.

Excerpts from political contributions to DA:NA
1. Labor Party, House of Representatives, Commonwealth Minister for Health
   The Hon. Neal Blewett, M.P.
   Opening address

It is important to get the issues in perspective. Public figures are much given to waxing eloquent and indignant on the evils of heroin and marijuana, and in the pursuit of moral uplift—or a rise in the party vote—are easily open to charges of hypocrisy. Heroin is not the biggest health problem in the area of drug abuse in this country. Alcohol abuse is. Many more of our young people will die or have their lives ruined as a result of alcohol-induced road accidents than will ever die of heroin overdoses or infected heroin needles. Much more hospitalisation in Australia will result from the ill effects of nicotine abuse than from marijuana abuse. And the misuse of pharmaceuticals, particularly barbiturates, occasions far more problems for doctors at present than cocaine.

This is not to argue that heroin, cocaine and marijuana do not pose potentially serious health problems for our society. It is merely to argue that they must be seen in the context of drug abuse more generally. Nor is it to argue that the culturally accepted drugs—alcohol, tobacco, barbiturates—should be made illegal; equally it is not to argue that the illegal drugs—heroin, cocaine, marijuana—be legalised. There are important historical, cultural and social considerations, which cannot simply be brushed aside, which explain why we are at our current position. What I am demanding is a proper perspective on drugs. It is a plea that if we are to avoid charges of hypocrisy, if we are not to render ourselves unbelievable to the young, then our perspective on drugs cannot narrowly concentrate on those that are illegal.

To have any prospect of success a national drug strategy needs to be both co-ordinated and multifaceted. At present the decision path chart on drug co-ordination looks somewhat like a complex version of one of those plans for a transistor radio. Unfortunately the sound emitted is far less coherent than that which emerges from a transistor radio. Therefore we have both to simplify and shorten the decision-making paths in any national drug strategy.

I turn now to a more specific issue—the treatment of heroin addiction. While there is no doubt a national preference for a drug-free treatment of heroin addicts, I found on my recent overseas tour a growing acceptance of other forms of treatment. The acceptance of drug maintenance programs for heroin addicts stems as much from the desire to limit the social impact of heroin abuse as to rescue the addict from the criminal milieu of the heroin trade.

It has been canvassed that heroin be made legally available to registered addicts in Australia. The advantages of this are obvious. It removes the addict from the trade in illegal heroin and from the petty criminal activity required to cover the costs of that addiction. But British experience over a long period of time suggests there are adverse consequences from making heroin legally available for the management of addicts. The necessity for three or four heroin injections a day imposes heavy costs if these are to be administered in health centres or surgeries under appropriate supervision. On the other hand, to supply addicts with two or three days' provision served too often simply to feed the illegal market with pure government- guaranteed heroin. Moreover, the supply of licit heroin involved maintaining a distribution and storage system with all its attendant security problems. I was not surprised to learn in discussions with Ministers and senior officials in the United Kingdom earlier this month that the use of licit heroin in the management of heroin addiction is being wound down.

What then can we offer the person physically dependent on illicit heroin? First of all I believe we must offer understanding, compassion and patience. Those of you who work or live with people dependent on heroin will immediately see behind those words—they will know how endlessly and purposefully irritating some patients and clients, some friends and relatives, can be. It can be difficult and demanding to maintain an effective helping and caring relationship. Work with drug-dependent people has much in common with caring for people with AIDS or incurable cancer—it requires that difficult combination of caring ability and emotional strength.

But caring alone, though essential, is usually not enough. Most people physically dependent on heroin require medical help, either as part of a detoxification program or as part of a longer treatment/ maintenance/ rehabilitation program; and in both of these they need an effective pharmacological alternative to heroin. Methadone is the alternative most used because it is effective when taken by mouth and its long-acting effects mean that it only needs to be taken once a day. In adequate dosages, methadone can offer many heroin addicts a real and effective alternative to dependence on illicit heroin with its attendant problems of uncertain supply, contaminated needles, contaminated cutting and uncertain dosage, the prostitution and criminal activity necessary to buy the heroin, potential conflict with the law, and the real possibilities of imprisonment. Small wonder that many trapped in the heroin vortex want to get out and believe that methadone treatment and maintenance is their only hope. We must seriously examine the possibility of expanding that alternative.

I am well aware of course that methadone is not in itself a cure for heroin addiction. But is does bring heroin addicts into a therapeutic relationship with a range of clinical staff who can help them to help themselves. It does enable them to escape the heroin sub-culture and often it enables many to return to employment and a normal social life.

Figure 4   Marijuana in the headlines (at right)

Marijuana — for and against

THE AUSTRALIAN
MARCH 6-7 1982

No room for hysteria in the cannabis debate

Those advocating decriminalisation of [marijuana] seem to ignore, even, the impressive evidence of its effects. By 1978, studies had been ... and more since, ... of which show ... potential harm ... use. Few have ... good to say about ...

A proposal for a major change to which people have become ... Government and the con... provokes resistance. ... reforms frequently borders ... the hysterical. The ... mendations of the Australian ... sation on Alcohol and Drug ... dence (AFADD) relating to the ... isation of marijuana are already ... ucing such a response.

... he report does not ... of marijuana is ... consequences a ... AFADD has conclud ... arijuana is so w ... xisting legal prohib ... eed for a better m ... what has become a f ...

According to 197 ... in the report, 16 per ... between the ages ... used marijuana, as ... those aged from ... cent of those bet ... and 20. These f ... that, whatever e ... provisions have ... have not ... becom ... pleas ...

concede is relatively harmless in comparison with drugs such as heroin, into contact with criminals who are willing to peddle anything provided there is money in it. There is no reliable evidence that the use of marijuana in itself induces the use of harder drugs, but it is apparent that there are links between the pushers of marijuana and the pedlars of heroin, and the latter are being presented with opportunities which result solely from marijuana's illegality.

LETTERS
Address letters to GPO Box 4162, Sydney, NSW 2001. Letters must have full name and address, although not necessarily for publication. Keep letters brief and include your telephone number for verification. Preference is given to typewritten letters. We reserve the right to edit them.

dies show it is psychologically and there are of physical withformance with usage of the only improves it.

...ys, it is worse ... or alcohol. ...hitis develops ...ths of heavy ...

this psychosis being permanent. Serious questions have been raised linking marijuana with birth defects, hormonal changes and decreased resistance to infections.

Countries w... of experience moves towa... We know enough to couraging (D...

prohibition ... annually costs ... of millions of ... basis for ... do our ... uate ...

readers that it is now the policy of the Queensland branch of the Australian Labor Party to decriminalise the possession and cultivation of marijuana for personal use. When I moved the motion to adopt this policy at the 1981 State Conference, I remember being pleasantly surprised at the virtually unanimous support it received.

Politics aside, the State Conference is made up of a wide cross-section of the Queensland community, including State and federal parliamentary leaders. The adoption of the policy, therefore, indicates 'widespread support in Queensland for the decriminalisation approach, as well as suggesting a widespread understanding that marijuana is a relatively ...mless drug.

A CONFIRMED and reformed smoker, I applau... recent expert co... report recommend decriminalisation marijuana.

Australian soc... fraught with h... double standard... hocus-pocus in its ... to drugs. M... dangerous? Wha... aspirin, tobacco a... hol!

Alcohol kills. Di... its effect on the fa... consumed imme... indirectly, by its ... those who kill and... our roads while ... influence — 3508 A... killed and 91,793 i... traffic accidents i... example (Year B... tralia 1981), and a ... tionate share of ... to alcohol.

Tobacco kills. ... U.S. Surgeon ... report points t... smoking as the ... preventable cause ... world-wide.

We deride wo... admiring those ... of their booze ... ers go u... ed as ... ...aces, ...

LEGALISE POT — REPORT

From BRUCE DOVER

CANBERRA. — Marijuana should be made legal, a group of prominent Australians say in a top level report.

Aus... They call for a governmental monopoly to... on marijuana in Australia with the Commonwealth Scientific and Industrial Research Organisation controlling lawful manufacture, quality and sales.

The report says the group believes possession, use and homegrown marijuana should be legal.

Warning

However, he pointed out that the report was only a discussion paper and ... the Australian Foundation on Alcoholism and Drug Dependence (AFADD).

The report said advertising would be restricted and health warnings similar to those imposed ... to discourage ... to be ... would also ...

Marijuana: Do you want it?

Pin-pointing the facts behind today's shock drugs rec...

By its very nature, the use, misuse or non use of marijuana is a highly contentious political and moral topic.

BY GRAHAM RICKNELL

Lega... drug... supp... urge...

The NSW Attorney-General, Mr Walker, said yester... day that the State Govern... ment had no intention of changing the law on marihuana.

Mr Walker said the Government had already firmly indicated that consideration of the matter was under consideration.

In ... the Australian Foundation on Alcoholism and Drug Dependence, and recommended that possession, use and homegrowing of marijuana be legalised.

A special committee including the chairman of the Law Reform Commission, Mr Justice Kirby, Sir David Bliss and the Australian Institute of Criminology of the Department of Crim... Univer...

Controversy over 'legal pot' report

CANBERRA — A major report recommending legalisation of marijuana has sparked immediate controversy.

From our Canberra Bureau

A group of prominent Australians is pressing the Federal Government and the communities to rebrace drug laws and attitudes

The group wants a public debate to get people in late so to what it calls so on marijuana as opposed to al cohol and narcotics

It also wants to bring attention to the industry of penal laws to cope with financial running of syndicates and police corruption.

The group's recommendations in a discussion paper on alcohol, cannabis and heroin sponsored by the Australian Foundation on Alcoholism and Drug Dependence.

The report was distributed last Monday for release this Monday, but the embargo was broken yesterday in the Sydney Telegraph — part of Mr Rupert Murdoch's News Ltd organisation.

The most well-known and influential member of the committee include the chairman of the Law Reform Commission Mr Justice Kirby, Tasmanian Liberal Senator Shirley Walters, the associate director of the Australian Institute of Criminology Mr David Biles, and former Queensland Police Commissioner Mr Ray Whitrod.

The group recommends that individuals should be allowed to grow marijuana for their own use but that all other production be prohibited.

It calls on the Government to control the manufacture and distribution to ensure a standard and uniform quality.

Profits would be an incentive to discourage black market activities but not so low as to boost sales and increase use.

The group suggests the CSIRO would be an appropriate body to make a feasibility study on a Government ...

Marijuana laws 'a stigma on citizens'

By PETER DWYER

A report on social policies and drugs in Australia had not recommended the immediate decriminalisation of marijuana, according to a member of the workshop which prepared it.

The Professor of Community Medicine at the University of Tasmania, Professor Narelle Lickiss, said in Hobart yesterday the recommendations concerning marijuana had been ...n out of context.

...controversial report was ... publicity for its re... ...ns on marijuana, ...sation and a ...ooly on its

..."icised the

The CANNABIS DEBATE

SELL GOLD, BUY MARIJUANA! SHARES

the call for legalisation of cannabis and the formation of a Government monopoly.

She said it was 'not 'edition and unpleas' to demand those measures knowing little of health effects of the organisation.

The paper says users of the drug should know but mothers use should be discouraged.

Mr Justice report, issued whether the drug is all through the th... He said a grou... otherwise law abid... had criminal records ... they used cannabis ...

He said Mr Dwyer los... since the laws when people were penalised for activities that did not compare with ... the control of the prop... any accepting the use of mari... huana on a level with alcohol and tobacco.

A former Prime Minister, Sir John Gorton, said the committee's findings were 'thoroughly right' and he also favored de...

...present, almost it... uation."

She said ...ously seen ... the fact ... were bi... using ...

P... th... p...

LAWS ON MARIHUAN... 'WON'T BE CHANGED'

A SHOCK report recommending that marihuan... legalised and under ... trol of the CSIR... slapped ...

...egalisation of marijuana urged

EY: The NSW Young ... Movement said yesterday ... recommendations for ... riminalisation of mari... possession and cultivation made by the Australian ... ion on Alcoholism and ... ependence did not go

decriminalisation without full legalisation were illogical.

The movement believed that the Commonwealth and State parliaments should introduce legislation to bring about the full legalisation of marijuana without further delay.

Mr Crawford said that the Pre...

...posals out of hand.

He said he was disappointed that the Leader of the Opposition, Mr Dowd, did not support decriminalisation but would attempt to persuade him to rethink his views.

Mr Dowd said yesterday that he would meet with Mr Crawford but

said ... y the ... on Al... Dependence , inter ... ipma the present r ... laws put on oth... biding citizens.

a matter of whet... of wider use of fu... gh decriminalis ... gh a price to pa...

2. **Labor Party, Senate Chairman of Caucus Committee on Community Health**
   Senator Rosemary Crowley
   An informal address

It is important for us to know how many people have devoted a fair amount of their lives and 'busted their guts' on behalf of people with drug and alcohol problems for the last God knows how many years in this country. It is not as though we have been doing nothing in Australia. Lots of very important things have been done and there are plenty of people in the community who are evidence, and olympic evidence, of the help they have received.

Definitions

We need to be very clear about what we mean when we talk about drugs. The licit drugs within this country really do have to be included in our deliberations. I don't suppose too many of us see aspirin as a drug of dependence, but aspirin has been a drug that has caused a great many problems.

For the women of Australia, a cup of tea, a Bex and a good lie down have been presented as a very useful and appropriate and moderate way to control difficulties in their lives. And quietly, they are poisoning their kidneys and themselves to death. The consequence is that we then have to invent renal machines in renal dialysis units and employ very expensive doctors and staff to look after those people with kidney disease. Then we run a campaign saying that people who take too much aspirin are rather naughty and at least failures in the coping business of this world.

Deliberations on drugs need to be comprehensive. The patterns of drug taking are not dissimilar if you go looking for the similarities. Are we examining drugs because they are illegal as currently defined, because they are associated with big money crime or because of the cost to the community—witness the cost consequences of aspirin excess, or the cost of human misery and suffering and exploitation—or all of these. We need to be clear!

Services

There is a very extensive variety of services of treatment and support and caring in the community. Such a variety of treatment services needs to be promoted and continued, and it is important that we have such a flexible range, providing the option for people that would best match their needs.

Some people do very well in withdrawal type houses. Some prefer the support of the community from something iike Alcoholics

Anonymous. Some people prefer a daily contact with a support person, others can manage very well as long as they know there is that person or that facility there they can drop in and see. Some places do much better in providing a package of treatment that continues after a withdrawal phase. Some people may prefer to manage their drug and alcohol problems by remaining in their community and being helped by their immediate community.

Care for carers
A lot of us can get caught up with trying to help patients not become dependent, not become defeated, not to give up. But we may in fact forget to provide for that same kind of energy for optimism amongst ourselves, the planners, amongst the people supporting the planners, the providers of care and the treaters. They need to be cared for too, and they need to care for themselves, so that they don't burn out or just quietly turn grey and depressed. As a corollary to this point, we have a lot of skilled workers, a lot of people who have learnt by living closely to drug-dependent and alcohol-dependent people. I think we need to look for their expertise as a source of wisdom for ourselves. Before we necessarily start courses in tertiary colleges or universities there is a lot of expertise that we can call on.

Advertising
We may have to be pluralist too in our approach to primary prevention or advertisement campaign. Talking about the ill effects of taking aspirin may result in people being appalled to discover the consequences. It is a reasonable guess that the people taking the aspirin don't see themselves as drug takers. They see themselves as moderately and responsibly medicating against the difficulties in their lives. A heroin campaign, however, would have a different focus. I don't suppose it would go along the lines that if your mate mainlines or shoots up in your house, don't let him drive!—as one drink driving advertisement in South Australia suggests as a way to prevent car accidents associated with alcohol.

Perhaps mothers are the cause of it all and we could prevent drugs in this world by doing away with mothers! More seriously, we do have to look at whether it is a parental problem or a parental contribution, we do have to look at whether unemployment is contributing, or whether in fact the problem is no worse than it was two thousand years ago. There are always problems associated with teenagers or the next generation and I urge caution about thinking we have a new problem in 1985, and ask whether things are not very different from 1935, or 1895.

3. Labor Party, House of Representatives, Member for Canberra Ms Ros Kelly, M.P.

I approach this seminar with a degree of cynicism—another meeting with what results?

Over the past ten years we have witnessed in Australia a plethora of Royal Commissions and Inquiries into Drug Trafficking and Abuse.

Enormous resources have been directed into these inquiries but with what result? There is no evidence that there is any decline in the extent of drug trafficking—all the evidence in fact points to an increase. There has been no massive breaking of organised crime networks, despite the fact that the names of the leaders of these networks are well known.

There are no detailed research statistics available in Australia to tell us about the extent of the drug problem, and most of all despite all our pious utterings of concern in this area only $2 million is expended per year under the National Drug Education Program.

Today we have the highest per capita consumption of alcohol in the English-speaking world and yet in discussions on drug abuse, the governing image of drug use and abuse in Australia is the association between illicit drugs and international crime syndicates, murder, and drug-crazed property theft.

There is absolutely no doubt that a coherent, national policy on drugs which our culture and its representatives deem to be illicit, is of vital importance. Of special attention here could be the strengthening of the Customs barrier, to make certain that crime does *not* pay.

I note that addiction workers in Canberra have in the main been excluded from your list of participants. Because this has been a matter of some concern to those workers, a drug abuse seminar was organised for the non- participants last Sunday. I want you all to know the general conclusions.

From the *lawyers* present came a call for the expansion of sentencing options with a greater emphasis on the counselling and treatment option.

Recovering addicts called for a first point of contact to be available outside office hours, and a variety of treatment and rehabilitation options.

Addiction workers primarily need ongoing funding and more help from trained workers. There are few training facilities in Australia, and no method of evaluation and accreditation of treatment programs.

Parents pointed out that the effects of addiction on the family can be catastrophic and like all others present they raised the need for widespread community education.

Everybody agreed that the problem won't go away by pretending it doesn't exist. The problem does exist, but very few people recognise symptoms of addiction, or have any idea about where to go for help and information.

My priorities for the National Campaign Against Drug Abuse are:

(a) that resources be put into the information action plan for a TV and print media campaign about the symptoms of addiction
(b) that rehabilitation and treatment workers have recognised training programs, and rehabilitation programs could be accredited as a pre-requisite to ongoing funding
(c) that distinctions be made between licit and illicit drugs so that respect for the law can be firmly re-established.

We have established the fact that as Australians we have a problem in the area of drug abuse. We have established some consensus on the need to ameliorate the problem. We can establish priorities for action ... it is time to get to work.

4. **Liberal Party, Senate, Past Commonwealth Minister for Health**
Senator The Hon. Peter Baume with Dr John Ellard

Public policies related to drug use in Australia are neither rational nor effective. If we are to help provide useful input to a national drug summit, then we must get the issues and the options right.

A national drug summit which looks only at problems of illicit drug use will fail to consider the bulk of Australia's drug problems.

A national summit which looks only at the means of limiting the supply of drugs will be doomed inevitably to be as unsuccessful as other similar conferences have been.

Drug use is part of our culture and part of most of our lives. We use drugs for adequate and proper reasons arising from our needs for relaxation, escape from tension, and as part of cultural heritage.

Total drug abstinence is not possible, it is even doubtful that it is desirable.

Any national policy which has as its goal the abolition of drug use is doomed to failure even before it has begun; any conference which highlights the effects of some drugs and ignores the greater adverse effects of other drugs will perpetuate what has been a sterile and a foolish approach to drug problems in this country.

If drug abstinence is not an option, then the national task is to determine the conditions under which drugs are used, and to devise realistic policies relating to their supply, to the extent of the demand for them, and towards reducing their adverse effects.

If drug use is inevitable and part of our society, then we need to accept, without being unduly emotional, that there will be casualties associated with the use (abuse) of drugs. This applies to the use of any drug. In the same way, we accept that motor vehicles are a necessary part of our existence even though they maim or kill many members of our society. There is no possible national strategy that will be without some casualties.

In Australia we have significant problems related to abuse of many drugs, but they are compounded by entrenched beliefs which lead us to deny the existence of some problems and to dramatise others.

Figures released by the Commonwealth Department of Health, based on the 1980 Census, estimate that of the 108 695 deaths recorded in that year 20 413 or 18.8 per cent were considered drug-related. Of the drug-related deaths almost 80 per cent were attributed to tobacco-related diseases, 17.55 per cent to alcohol use and 3.3 per cent were linked to other drugs. This figure, 3.3 per cent, includes accidental deaths (e.g. with children) and deliberate self-poisoning with sedatives. Deaths from street drugs were but a part of that small portion.

Inevitably this situation will bring any government into conflict with commercial interests whose goal is the increased use of their own products and sooner or later some government will need to be more courageous to do this in the national interest. It will have to negotiate new arrangements and undertakings with the marketers of legal drugs, even including arrangements to their commercial detriment.

In relation to illegal substances, much of the problem facing society is a consequence of the measures society itself has taken trying to limit the supply of the substances. We ignore the fact that there are costs and benefits associated with anything we do. We seem to have ignored completely the costs of the prohibition era in the United States. These costs included the emergence of exactly the same ruthless and effective criminal marketing network as we have made inevitable in our country to satisfy a market for certain substances.

Let it be clear that we are not advocating here the legalisation of the use of illicit substances.

Addiction *is* a major crisis for anyone. But we all know that it is possible for many addicts to live successful, productive, useful and relatively happy lives, if they have an assured supply of the substance. This is the basis of methadone maintenance programs.

There is a conspiracy of silence or indifference about the drug needs and the drug dependence of the middle-aged mainstream population. There is a corresponding conspiracy of outrage about the drug use of the young where it differs from that of older established Australians.

The press plays its part by giving undue emphasis to the sensational aspects of drug misuse and ignoring most of the grinding, continuing misery and illness and death which follow the use of socially accepted drugs.

We must make it possible for people to discuss the wide spectrum of drug use problems without the sense of threat that inhibits such an examination today. There is an urgent need to reassure people and to make them less frightened.

Does society see the fix they're in?

The considerable concern about drug use in our society is exemplified in the many Royal Commissions and Parliamentary Inquiries held since 1970; the calling of submissions for the 1985 National Campaign Against Drug Abuse by our present Minister for Health; the 507 responses to that call from concerned members of the public; the calling of a national workshop on drugs in Canberra; and the massive Australia-wide media coverage of these events.

The national workshop (DA:NA) attracted a significant amount of coverage around Australia by the media. The newspaper headlines in Figure 5 tell the story of the social issues involved, and the social attitudes at the time.

Newspaper cuttings of even one event, as in Figure 5, illustrate the fixed focus of different views and social interests. There may be no need to remove our old spectacles if the expectations of society, or significant elements of it, match the principles, policies and actions of any of the restricted views. In fact, it can be argued that real development will only occur as a result of one of the single visions, which turns out to be the most acceptable of all. But when the expectations are not being met, the glasses need removing. When politicians of all parties can agree on an issue, the glasses are coming off, and a common view is emerging.

A useful story to conclude this chapter comes from the British atomic tests in the South Australian desert thirty years ago. One of the bombs exploded was called TOTEM 1. On 24 April 1985, the McClelland Royal Commission sought evidence of past harm from Aboriginal inhabitants of the area. This was complicated because the very word 'death' in the language of that area is taboo; not even the names of those who died at that time, or since, could be mentioned. This dramatises the extent to which groups in society when confronted by conflicting value positions are often unable to translate those problems into mutually comprehensible terms.

Figure 5   Drugs in the headlines (see over)

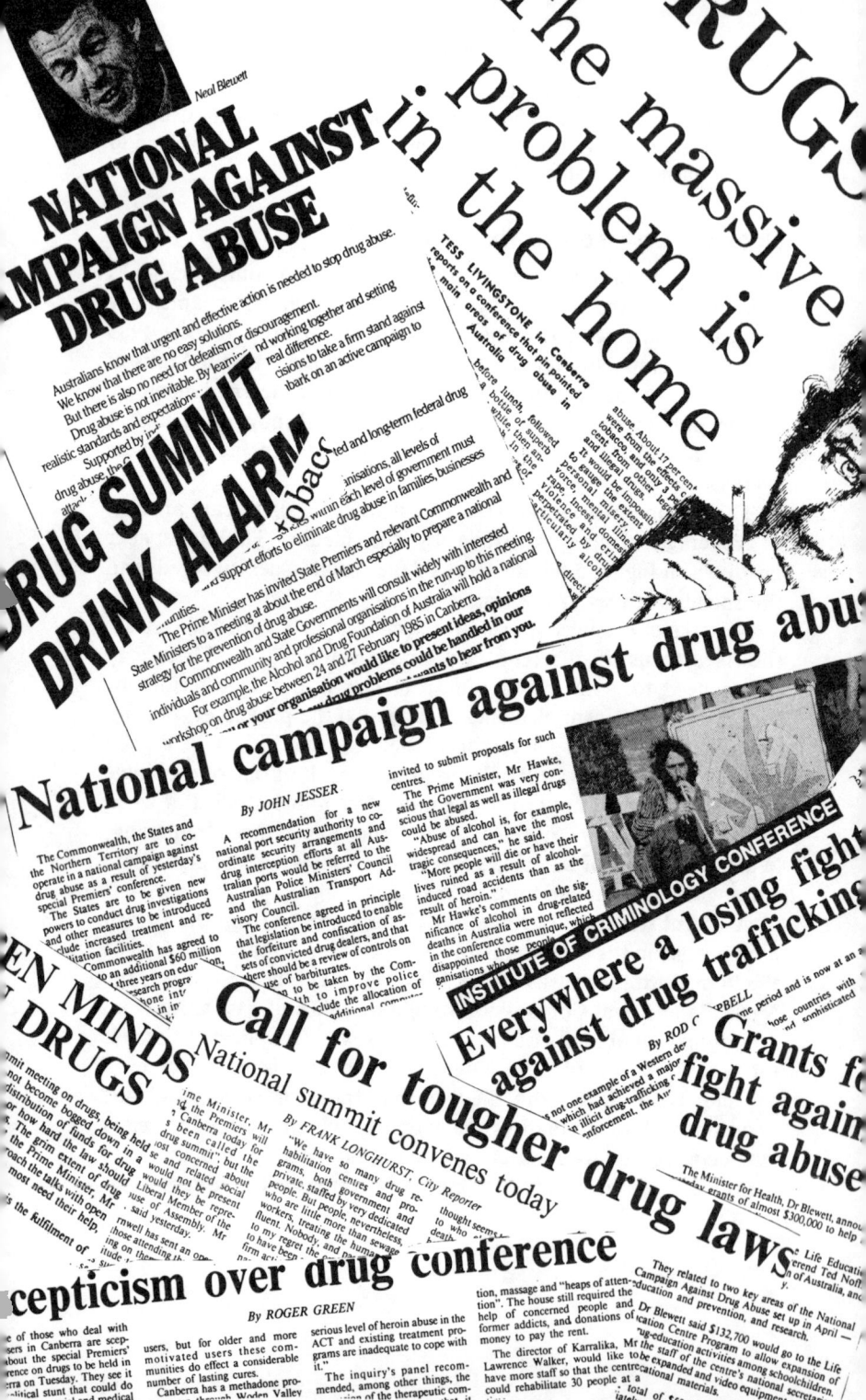

3
Drug Policy, Politics And Values

What is policy?

Policy is a consensus on the ideas that form the basis of action. As Titmuss has said (page 23), 'It is the principles which govern action directed towards given ends'. Policy statements are especially necessary when a society needs to change, and any co-ordinated approach to an issue requires such an overall direction. Government is often criticised for acting in kneejerk responses to changing events. To some, this is pragmatism, but what it really demonstrates is a lack of policy without which the lasting resolution of problems cannot occur.

Policy is not merely an abstract governmental phenomenon. It is needed and used in everyday life. The purchase of a house is, for most of us, the biggest investment of our lives—it is not undertaken without care and thought. What that purchase really amounts to is action on a policy decision about the kind of lifestyle and future we want. On a lower level, the purchase of the weekly groceries is almost done without thinking. But behind it is often a complex policy which has decided the elements of a healthy diet: the balance of food groups, the proportion to be spent on necessities and luxuries, the amount to be spent and so on.

It seems obvious that policy is important. All too often it is overlooked. And where policy decisions are made, they often deal only with means and not ends. Policy on means does affect ends; but if this happens without the ends being properly considered, the result is a society that develops as if by accident. Thus the Special Premiers' Conference on Drugs produced a policy on methadone, but methadone is not an end in itself; it is a means and a means to ends that have not yet been properly considered. We simply do not know enough to predict the result of continued use of methadone as the preferred treatment for heroin addiction in this country.

Will we have a large number of socially accepted addicts? A group of trapped, totally dependent individuals? No decline in the number of drug-addicted people? An escape hatch to a drug-free life? Perhaps even a society in which the misfits are expected to spend their lives passive, powerless and under control? These are the scenarios, and it is clear that the ends of means-policies must be evaluated and ends-policies carefully considered, if the risks above are to be avoided. We can also see that policy choices of either ends or means do not just solve problems, in some cases they also create problems. All policies have costs as well as benefits. For example, the very illegality of heroin inevitably increases the use of unsterile needles and so adds to the risk of death by hepatitis and AIDS. This has serious implications for strategies of control, and whether heroin should therefore be legalised is a serious proposition for policy makers.

What then must a social policy on drugs consider? This chapter deals with the development of realistic aims for drug use in society and the establishment of priorities. The question of priorities has twofold relevance: first, in deciding on the importance of the distinction between illegal and legal drugs; second, in deciding upon what approach to take in tackling problems of drug abuse. Here the issues raised in Chapter 2 become important in recognising the many views and values that abound, and the social and historical variables which create certain fixed perspectives. In deciding how to approach drug issues in Australia at the moment there is a tendency to adopt and stick to one of the four established attitudes of control, treatment, education and social change, with the last one usually relegated to the too hard basket.

Beliefs and policy

Why is there this entrenchment of interests in the policies that are taken on drug issues? It is because the attitudes of policy makers are dependent upon the same underlying beliefs and values that we all share. The world in the head of each of us, which underlies and controls all our actions and feelings, especially dominates in areas such as policy questions, where ideas are being formulated. The world in our heads allows us to make sense of the chaos in the universe but it also creates dogmatism and stops us from seeing that one man's totem is another's taboo. This applies not only to writers on ideologies. Philosophy is not the sole preserve of philosophers, nor politics of politicians, any more than dietitians are the only people with a diet.

The writers of this book have not been able to avoid these belief structure underpinnings any more than the rest of society has. It is important to appreciate, however, the role that these play in formulating responses to drug use and abuse. We believe that there is no objective 'answer' to the issues of possession of marijuana, methadone maintenance or drug education. The approach that is taken on these matters depends on the beliefs of the decision makers. We do believe that the results of a policy can, however, be stringently evaluated.

We carry in our minds an image of the kind of society that we desire, formulated by individuals and communities, and developed and nurtured in organisations such as churches and schools. Often, however, such images remain largely unexpressed. The gap between politics, which is seen as being pragmatic, and people's understanding of the world, which is seen in terms of deepest feelings and identity, is difficult to bridge in words. Moreover, those who depend strongly on practical matters on one hand and intuition on the other often do not trust each other.

Table 6 attempts to pinpoint the different world-views or political perspectives that exist, broadly, in Australia today, and to indicate the effect that these views have on drug policy. Although what is presented is in terms of *policy*, it should be appreciated that they can be interpreted in any or all of the three *levels of action* (policy, strategies and action plans), the framework for which is outlined in Figures 3 and 4. Political beliefs decide not only policy but *strategies and action plans* too. Moreover, political views arise out of their *social context* and the social context can, in its turn, be altered by political action.

We have tried to provide some guideposts, with familiar examples, to the way political positions, our everyday attitudes, and our deep beliefs about the world fit together as 'drug policy'. Table 6 uses some metaphors and parables to link some of our society's most powerful totems to policy formulation.

Table 6
Politics, values and policy

Politics	Desired society	Values	Drug policy
		Paddle your own canoe	
1. Laissez faire	Anarchy	As few restrictions on human behaviour as possible.	No legal control over drugs.
		Faith in human ability to make rational, self-preserving choices.	Limited treatment facilities or support mechanisms.
		No man is an island	
2. Humanist	Socialist democracy	Concerned not to impose moral values.	Limited legal controls.
		Concern for pragmatic human needs.	More willing to provide treatment and support.
		Man overboard	
3. Existential	Individualist	Sees ultimate significance in the individual's response to circumstances. Individual must take responsibility for his own actions.	Control and treatment are seen as consequences of individual action, i.e. they are taken as 'given' but are not useful avenues for intervention. Emphasis on counselling, psychodrama and other measures directed at individual change.
		Noah's ark	
4. Social contract	Liberal democracy	The government has power to rule, by consent of the governed.	Control measures are seen as a valid expression of the will of the majority.
		In return for which, the public is given prosperity and benefits.	The other side of the contract is the provision of adequate treatment facilities, and the education of children to discourage drug abuse and encourage social responsibility.

DRUG POLICY, POLITICS AND VALUES

The Captain of the ship

5. Neo-conservative	Corporate state dictatorship or state capitalism	The government is the preserver of the status quo. Emphasis on moral values as seen by rulers.	Control measures are justified as a deterrent and punishment. More sympathetic measures are rejected as drug abuse is seen as being deviant.

Walking on the water

6. Theist	One open to external direction (expressed through human institutions)	The existence of a supreme authority (god). A morality created by God and unchanging.	Control measurers may be valid to protect an irresponsible drift in moral values. The approach is often sympathetic to measures designed to reform, e.g. by counselling, education, peer group/family prevention.
		Strong mandate for social change to bring about a certain vision of society (spiritual).	Social change may be an acceptable way to change drug use habits, depending on the current position of the church in society.

A tide in the affairs of men

7. Communist	Communist or socialist	Conflict and revolution are an inevitable and desirable part of human progress, to bring about a certain vision of society (material).	Individual change, treatment and control are all inadequate because they seek to adjust the individual to an imperfect society. Drug abuse is an active element in bringing about, and can only be redressed by, far-reaching social change.
		Societal behaviour can be explained in terms of class conflict and economic alienation.	Drug use is merely one symptom of alienation and oppression. Any intervention which does not see this is doomed to failure.

Note: these clear-cut lines are, in the real world, fuzzy and overlapping.

The situation outlined in Table 6 is further confounded because present political parties (in the sense of formal politics) are often a contradictory mix of these moral viewpoints (as most of our own decisions are). Thus the Liberal Party can be recognised as some sort of mix betweeen positions 1, 4 and 6 in Table 6. The latter two views dominate in the area of drugs, but the extent to which control measures are justified is tempered by the party's commitment to the first. This is especially so in the area of economic controls—for example, the extent to which the advertising of licit drugs should be limited—since the philosophy of economic laissez faire is still strong. Similarly, the Labor Party can be seen as a mix of 2, 4 and 7. In the area of drugs, humanism seems to prevail but this is not so in many other areas of government policy. For example, Labor governments have not been reluctant to apply legal controls to areas such as trade practices. Moreover, the enormous range of views in the Labor Party makes it impossible to define one clear value position.

The existence of apparently contradictory views side by side is not the sole privilege of political parties. Within many organised churches there is a great tension between the radical socialist element pressing for social change, and the neo-conservative element protecting and being protected by the status quo. The classic example of this is the current conflict between parts of the Catholic Church in South America.

That our view of society and the values we hold underpin our opinions of drug use has been shown by considering the way policy choices are affected by political values. Politics in this broad sense is influential on a practical level too. For example, it affects:

(a) The definition of the problem. A conservative viewpoint may be unwilling to include licit drugs as part of the 'drug abuse problem'.

(b) The priority given to various techniques of drug help. Those who accept the guidance of higher authority (religious or governmental) are more likely to accept assessment and diversion to compulsory treatment or to some kinds of therapeutic communities.

(c) Evaluation of a strategy or an action. The issue of what constitutes success is governed by political values. For those who see use of a drug as deviant or aberrant, nothing less than a totally drug-free outcome will be acceptable. The conflict over the validity of methadone maintenance is largely political, not technical.

Thus the political assumptions of an individual or community do not just govern what consequences are desired. They also govern what strategies and action are considered. Political constraints operate as structural impediments in the implementation of policy.

At government level

Government philosophy restricts and governs possible courses of action. Thus the Baume report recommended far-reaching changes in our approach to licit drugs. The then Commonwealth Government's (1980) philosophy of free enterprise restricted its ability to implement many of the recommendations. Further, the government's political concern with fiscal management led it to reject considering excise levels of alcohol and tobacco in anything other than 'a budgetary context'. Community pressure for some sort of action, however, forced the government to channel resources into politically acceptable fields, such as the National Drug Education Program. Similarly, the Sackville Commission (1979) recommended partial legalisation of cannabis. Almost immediately, the South Australian Government changed, and buried not merely the recommendation but the whole report.

At a social level

The broad political values of the society also limit what can be done. Measures will fail if community support is not forthcoming. In addition, any government is unlikely to act in a way which will lose it many votes. The effect of closing down the alcohol industry, on the economy and on unemployment, would be such that one cannot imagine a government conceiving such a measure; and yet we are near to considering closing down the tobacco industry in this country.

At a community level

There is no such thing as one monolithic community; our society is composed of many small communities—ethnic, professional, regional and so on. Some of these communities have great power and can effectively constrain government action. State and Federal bureaucracies, for example, are entrenched power bases able to stifle initiatives which threaten them. Any move aimed at allowing Federal Police to take over State responsibilities in the area of drug trafficking would meet with such resistance as to make its implementation highly impractical. Baume has commented that the surest way to have a recommendation ignored is to advocate the disbanding of jobs or areas of responsibility.

Community reaction to any widespread legalisation of illicit narcotics is likely to be so adverse that such an action would not be viable at least in the short term. Social context, then, sets the parameters for strategies, and so for viable policies.

At a professional level
Professional communities such as doctors are strongly placed to resist government intrusion; the present conflict over Medicare is an example of that. Many people argue that one of the main problems of drug abuse is the way in which we have been educated to believe that every problem has a chemical solution, and every heartache its soluble white tablet. Any attempt to implement a policy aimed at reducing these perspectives is likely to meet great hostility from doctors and drug companies. In a very real sense, professional organisations and special interest groups form political limits on potential action. Sax, in his history of health care in Australia, gives us chapter and verse for this.

At the level of everyday language
The use of language is very powerful in political terms because it triggers images within a strongly held framework of beliefs. Sometimes the use of these triggers is unconscious, and sometimes deliberate. The invoking of 'druggies', or 'the family', or 'national pride', especially by the mass media as described by Bell and Windschuttle, sets off whole trains of feeling and thought. The consequences of these trains of thought more often than not are then left to stand by themselves unexamined and unquestioned. We hope that Figure 11 can be used as a practical aid to identify the framework of beliefs behind such thought processes, and to identify for readers where they stand, where they wish to end up, and how to understand other viewpoints.

Priorities of approach

It is being recognised that stopping drug use is neither possible nor desirable. For example, prohibition of alcohol was partially successful in USA, but the social costs proved unacceptable.

The first question in deciding policy issues therefore must be, to what extent is society entitled to control individuals' drug use? It is argued that the control of mood-altering drugs is society's moral duty. Considering the widespread use of alcohol, tobacco, coffee and tea in our society, this stance is very simplistic. Moreover the history of laws introduced to enforce morality is a sorry one, riddled with social disharmony. Policy makers must never lose sight of the fact that people use drugs because they fulfil a need. Drug use for good or ill is a coping mechanism.

A libertarian society would not control drugs at all, but neither would it provide treatment or support. Australia is not such a society. Nevertheless, in Australia civil liberties are valued and the extent of social interference must be carefully delimited. Le Dain and Sackville conclude that policy must be concerned with the harmful consequences of drug use. Different drugs have different levels at which use is harmful to public safety and community health and welfare. Policies need to be tailored accordingly. Most of the major inquiries, summarised in Table 1, have taken this position.

An approach aimed at limiting harmful consequences will not be restricted to controls over drug use only when it causes harm. First, young people may need to be specially protected. Second, as Ledermann has established, controls over total consumption have been shown to affect the number of problem users and drug-dependent persons. But in implementing this 'consumption model' consideration should be given to the extent to which the majority should be controlled because of the immoderate habits of a few.

Concern in the community is largely directed towards the use of illicit drugs. This false distinction has led, for example, to an emotive concern over cannabis which seems to some out of proportion to its use and dangers. It has also affected funding priorities and the development of laws. For example, in the ACT it is not an offence to drive while adversely affected by drugs such as Serepax, or anti-histamines. The courts have held that such products are not within the meaning of the word 'drug' in the Ordinance. The distinction suggests that illicit drugs are always more harmful than licit drugs and that all illicit drugs are equally dangerous. These assumptions are incorrect as the review of data in Chapter 4 will show. A rational policy must deal with the real areas of concern, regardless of the line of legality drawn by historical happenstance.

Nevertheless the distinction is not totally irrelevant. First, it limits viable strategies—a move to make alcohol illegal is impracticable, but a move to keep cannabis illegal is not. Furthermore, the context of use dictates suitable strategies. Alcohol, by virtue of its legality, is accepted and resultant problems are largely denied. Suitable strategies may be significantly different from those relating to illicit drugs. Thus, while the media and education strategies related to tobacco may have much to teach how we approach drug education generally, the success of a campaign in one area does not necessarily indicate its success elsewhere. Moreover, the tenets behind, for example, the trend towards prohibition of smoking in many public areas need to be questioned before they are applied to other drugs.

In Table 2 and Chapter 2 we drew on Helen Nowlis's work to outline and discuss the four major ways of seeing drug use, and described how these approaches are equivalent to coloured spectacles by which individuals and societies view drug use and abuse. At this historical moment, our society seems to be picking up and putting down spectacles indiscriminately. It is recognised that considered policy choices can and should be made. In order to make informed choices, it is essential that the implications of all the options are understood. Unfortunately, our specialised era tends to favour single avenues of response and single sets of spectacles. A summary of the presently established *ways of seeing* follows (see Table 7).

The *moral/legal* approach seeks to keep drugs away from people and primarily uses legal, ethical and religious controls to achieve its objectives. It sees the substance as the active component and people as passive victims, made so through ignorance or deviance. One problem with this approach is that it assumes that if you control the supply of a drug demand will dry up. Evidence of drug trafficking, however, indicates that once a market is established, if there is a demand, there will be people willing to take the risks of supply. In this approach, both supply and demand are assumed to be dangers to society.

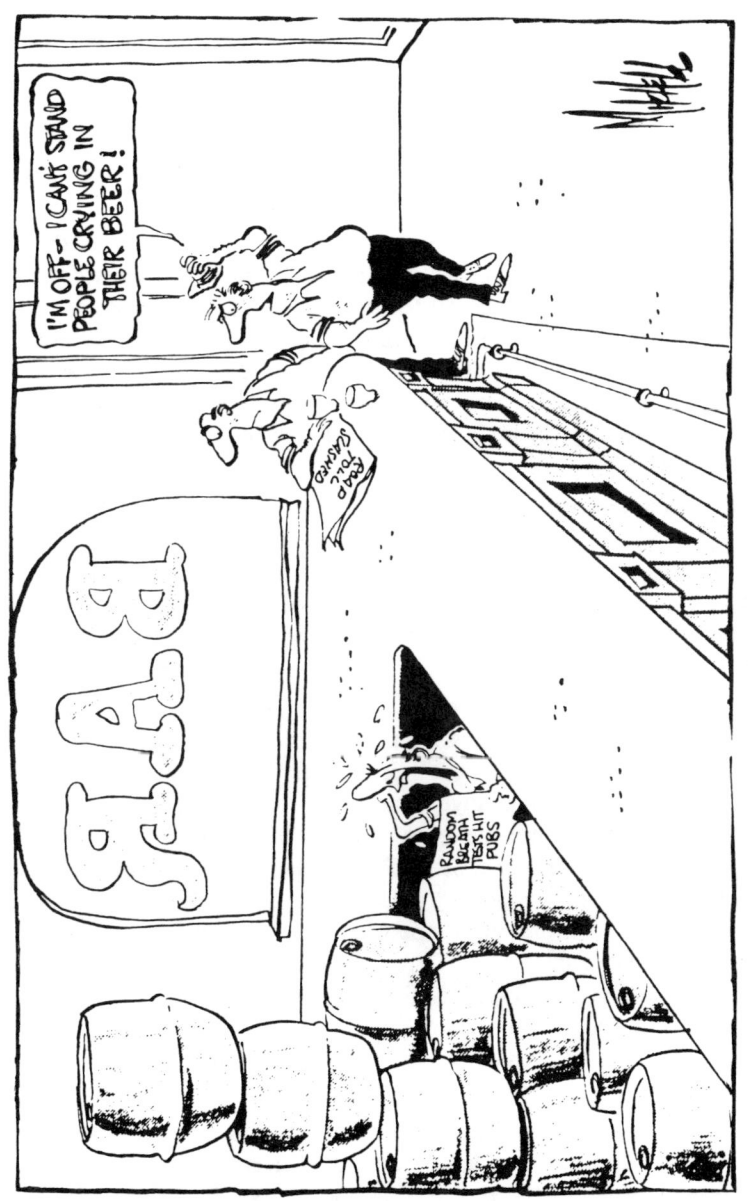

Cartoon by Mitchell, reprinted by permission of the artist, from *Australian*, 28 December 1982.

In the classic *public health* approach drug abuse is seen as a 'disease' that requires suitable treatment. This approach reflects the clinical treatment viewpoint. Unlike the previous model, it does not distinguish between licit and illicit drugs. It too, however, treats the user as a passive recipient of drugs, but in this case needing medical help. It therefore assumes that users are always in need of treatment. But using drugs, unlike mumps, is an active response to one's environment and users often do not want to be cured.

The *psycho-social* approach emphasises the individual as the active component. It investigates the motivation for drug use, in order to minimise the demand for drugs. It assumes that demand controls supply. The policy response using this approach will not be drug specific. As Baume said, it sees the 'drug problem' as a 'people problem'. The person is seen as responsible for his or her own drug-taking behaviour, and as ready to help change behaviour.

The *socio-cultural* approach sees drug use as gaining its meaning from the way in which a society defines and responds to use and users. For example, poverty, isolation, and unemployment are primary points of intervention. The origin of drug use is seen as the social setting and the individual actor can be either an independent actor or powerless within that setting.

In Table 7 these four approaches can be tied into the levels and avenues of response discussed in Chapter 1. It is important to recognise that each of these approaches has implications for control, treatment and change measures. Professional training and practice classically impose only one of these modes, and the matched avenues of response in Table 7 become railroad tracks. Ideally, any way of seeing drug use should draw on all four avenues of response. The moral/legal approach, for example, may favour legal controls, but it also permits a consideration of suitable treatment and prevention strategies. On the other hand, the socio-cultural way of seeing, while emphasising the need for social change, can also be used to develop control, treatment or education measures.

As Table 7 shows, the four approaches fall naturally into a dichotomy. The first two approaches see drugs as problems to be eradicated, whereas the last two see them largely as needs of the individual or the society.

DRUG POLICY, POLITICS AND VALUES 57

Table 7
Framework for drug issues 3 : policy analysis—a binary view

	AVENUES OF APPROACH			
			PREVENTION	
	Control	Treatment	Education	Social change
Policy				
Social context				
Strategy				
Action				
Ways of seeing	Moral/ legal	Public health	Psycho-social	Socio-cultural
Drugs are seen as	A PROBLEM FOR SOCIETY		OR A FUNCTION OF SOCIETY	

LEVELS OF ACTION

In recent years, policy analysts have favoured the psycho-social approach and consequently recommend strategies involving life skills and stress management. Front-line workers from any of the ways of seeing the problem are often restricted in the field to only control and treatment as avenues of response. The difficulty with a socio-cultural approach is that the community thinks nothing is being done about the 'problems' themselves, and demands a problem-centred approach. Drew et al. have argued that the community's concern over drugs is not related to fear about their effect on national security, increased crime, costs to the economy, health and so on; rather, many people are using 'drugs' as a scapegoat for more difficult underlying social problems and conflicts which are too painful to tackle.

Question: What would you do about glue sniffing in a New South Wales country town? Would banning glue help?

4
Effects And Extent Of Drug Use

Effects of drug use

Drugs can be natural or synthetic. They may be produced in laboratories or factories, sold over the counter with or without a prescription, for mood modifying or curative properties, grown in the garden or found in the bush. Some are only obtainable on the black market, and some are presently defined as illegal, although their status has little to do with their potential for harm. Drugs include powders, pills, gases, liquids and crystals and they are swallowed, drunk, inserted, injected, sniffed or inhaled. What they all have in common is that they are chemical substances with the ability to alter the physical and/or psychological state of the body. Used judiciously, many can be beneficial; misused they all have the potential for harm or death.

Broadly speaking there are three major types of drug. Depressants decrease the rate of normal bodily functions by slowing down the activity of the central nervous system, producing slower motor reactions, heart and breathing rates, and feelings of calmness, relaxation, stupor or drug sleep. Stimulants speed up the activity of the central nervous system, giving increased heart and breathing rates and a general state of arousal. Psychedelics may stimulate or depress, but the main effect is to distort perception and the thinking processes in a way which produces auditory, tactile and/or visual hallucinations.

Tabulated details of the most commonly abused chemical substances follow in Table 8. First we look briefly at the few things which can be said of all drugs.

Method of administration
The method of administration affects the speed with which a reaction will be obtained. Thus, sniffing, inhalation, suppositories and intravenous injections will generally have a much faster effect than from taking a drug by mouth or applying it to the skin. The digestive tract and epidermis have strong protective properties on behalf of their inhabitant, and select, extract or block many substances which have been taken orally or painted on. Other means of entry not only short circuit biological safeguards; their use is socially taboo, except through the totemised medical staff. Their use thus removes a drug user further from social acceptability.

Distribution
The distribution of a drug in the body varies considerably depending on its type. Some, such as alcohol, dissolve readily in liquids, others bind to fat or are attracted to particular parts of the body such as the bones. Some are prevented from entering parts of the body because of cellular barriers while others, like alcohol, are uniformly distributed throughout most areas of the body.

Metabolism
Once in the body a drug may be chemically altered, usually by the liver. During this process of metabolism, it may be made more active, like cortisone, or inactivated, like propranolol, or left in its original state, like digoxin. On repeated exposure to some drugs, the drug change process speeds up so that the drug is either rendered inactive faster, as with barbiturates, or its effects occur faster and are intensified, depending on the type of drug.

Drugs are excreted either through the kidneys (in urine), the intestine (in faeces), the lungs (in breath), skin (in sweat), mouth (in saliva) or through the breasts (in lactation). Rate of elimination varies enormously depending on the drug dose, mode of administration, weight, sex and age. It can take from minutes to weeks. A middie of beer, for example, takes about one hour to clear from the body, while cannabis lingers for many days.

Dosage
The amount required to obtain a desired effect varies between individuals. For many drugs, effective doses are determined by

factors such as weight and age. However, there are exceptions and some individual reactions can be totally unpredictable. We have little (formal) information about dosages for the non-medical products such as marijuana and the inhalants and it is possible, for example, for a novice sniffer to go into shock and die while others can continue for years.

The state of the individual, including health and time since the last meal, can also affect the reaction to a particular dose, as can state of mind and the existing social circumstances. The effects of marijuana can vary according to the user's expectations, while drinking alcohol can be a stimulating or depressing experience, depending on the circumstances in which it is taken.

An increase in dosage will at first produce an increase in effect, but after that threshold has been reached, increases in dosage will have little or no effect, apart from increasing side effects, until the lethal point is reached. The frequency with which a dose is administered also affects the chances of developing tolerance to the drug.

Tolerance
With continuing use of some drugs such as alcohol and narcotics tolerance may occur, so that the dose and frequency of administration have to be increased in order to obtain the original effect. Cross-tolerance can also occur when the tolerance developed for one drug works for another, as with heroin and methadone, and the need for a different anaesthetic dose for an alcoholic patient. Another type of cross-tolerance occurs in which the rate of tolerance varies for different effects of the same drug, as, for instance, its sedative and respiratory depressant effect. With LSD and some other hallucinogens, however, repeated doses over a few days appear to produce no increase or decrease in effect.

Dependence
It is possible to be physically and/or psychologically dependent on a drug, such as with physical and psychological dependence on smoking and psychological dependence on amphetamines.

A person is said to be physically dependent on a drug if withdrawal symptoms appear when the use of the drug is stopped. Such a state is a period of chemical readjustment for the body with characteristic symptoms occurring according to the type of drug.

Such dependence-producing drugs include alcohol, nicotine, barbiturates and narcotics.

Psychological dependence is said to occur when, on ceasing the use of the drug, the individual has a strong craving to continue in the drugged state because it enhances pleasurable feelings and coping ability. Effects of withdrawal from the most commonly abused drugs are listed in Table 8.

The World Health Organization (1982) defines drug dependence as a state in which self-administered drugs cause damage to self or society. Terms such as 'alcoholic' and 'addict' have been commonly used in the past, often with strong moral overtones. It is preferable to refer to a person being (physically or psychologically) *dependent* on a drug.

Side effects
All drugs have more than one effect on the body. Some of the unintended effects are potentially harmful, some are of little consequence and some are unnoticed, and so unknown. In medical care, benefits of use have to be weighed against disadvantages, as with pain-relieving drugs which can cause hearing disturbances. Caffeine stimulates urine production; smoking cigarettes assists relaxation but causes respiratory disease; heroin reduces pain in cancer patients but produces dependence (for the terminally ill, when dependence is irrelevant, modern synthetic drugs are considered adequate). Almost all drugs are taken for both physical and emotional effects. The physical effects, both pleasurable and harmful, are described in Table 8; the background to the emotional effects is described under the themes of social context and policy.

The effects of drugs on the foetus and newborn can be described under three headings: unknown, suspect and definitely harmful. Drugs in general cross the human placenta with ease. In many cases the effect of a drug on the foetus is unknown, as with Datura, cocaine and paracetamol. In some cases the evidence about their dangers is conflicting, as for instance with LSD, aspirin, caffeine and cannabis. In other cases there is definite proof of mild to severe harm, as with alcohol, nicotine, amphetamines and PCP. Given such potential risk to the health of the infant, it is usually recommended that the use of all drugs in pregnancy be avoided, unless the expected medical benefit appears to outweigh the risk.

Table 8
Most commonly abused chemical substances in Australia in 1985

PSYCHEDELICS (Hallucinogens)

Drug	Common or trade name	Immediate effects	Harmful long-term effects (risk)	Withdrawal effects	Legal status	Use and appeal
Lysergic acid diethylamide	'LSD' 'Acid'	Variable from mood changes through to florid hallucinatory experiences. (1)	May lead to flashback experiences or psychotic reaction. (1)	None.	Illegal, prohibited substance except for Datura and other plants.	Prevalence of use varies according to fads. Used mostly by the young, especially polydrug users.
Phencyclidine (PCP)	'Angel dust'					
Mescaline	'Mescal buttons' 'Peyote'	Some 'trips' are caused by amalgams of hallucinogens and cocaine or amphetamine and are less predictable.				Appealing in its so-called 'consciousness expanding effect', and its use as a 'chemical educator'. (except Datura).
4 Methol-2, 5 dimethoxy-amphetamine (DOM)	'STP'					
Datura and other plants	'Devil's trumpet' 'Magic mushrooms'					

Table 8 (continued)

Drug	Common or trade name	Immediate effects	Harmful long-term effects (risk)	Withdrawal effects	Legal status	Use and appeal
STIMULANTS						
Nicotine	As in cigarettes, cigars, pipes and nicotine chewing gum	Increase in heart rate and blood pressure; central nervous system stimulated. (2)	Lung cancer, mouth cancer, respiratory disease, especially emphysema and bronchitis; heart attack, poor circulation. (2)	Psychological and physiological dependence; headaches, cravings, irritability, bronchitis symptoms, nausea, increased appetite, palpitations, constipation. (2)	Sale of tobacco products illegal for under 16 years, also becoming illegal to use in some public places. Nicotine gum legally available on prescription only.	Increasing public disapproval and decrease in use amongst adults, but increase in use amongst young women. Provides stimulant and stress-coping mechanism, also oral gratification.
Caffeine (and similar substances)	As in tea, coffee, cocoa, cola drinks, chocolate, No-doze tablets	Increased alertness, heart rate, breathing, urine production, stomach secretions. (3)	Stomach ulcers, possibly contributes to risk of heart disease, bladder or kidney cancer. (3)	Mild to severe psychological and physical dependence, headaches, irritability, anxiety. (3)	Legal.	Widespread use and acceptance. Provides stimulant effect, oral gratification and acts as social lubricant.

EFFECTS AND EXTENT OF DRUG USE

Phenylpropanolamine	Many cough, cold, and compound preparations	Raised blood pressure, heart rate, risk of stroke. Anxiety, nervousness, insomnia, muscle tremors, fits, altered mental state, nausea, vomiting, hallucinations. Relaxes bronchioles. (4)	Raised blood pressure. Little information available. (1)	Little information available. Rebound nasal stuffiness. (4)	Legal. Prescription only except small amounts in over the counter (OTC) compound preparations.	Used by different subgroups depending on the substance, but frequently by young people. Used for stimulant effect.
Pseudoephedrine	Sudafed				Legal. Available through pharmacies only.	
Ephedrine	Ephedrine				Legal. Available through pharmacies only.	
Amphetamines	'Beanies' 'Uppers' 'Speed'	Reduced appetite, increased respiration, heart function and blood pressure, prolonged concentration, insomnia, euphoria. (2)	Amphetamine psychosis, violence, malnutrition, depression, lethargy, risks associated with high blood pressure. (2)	Psychological dependence. (2)	Legal. Prescription only. However, prescriber has to first obtain authority from State Health Authority (Medical Officer of Health) for prescribing. Only allowed for a few specific conditions.	Some popularity amongst adolescents and young adults.
Amphetamine sulphate	Benzedrine					Also occupational use, e.g. drivers.
Dexamphetamine sulphate	Dexedrine					Appealing in its effect of supposedly prolonging concentration and wakefulness.
Methylamphetamine	Desoxyn					

(Methylphenidate, e.g. Ritalin, has similar effects)

Table 8 (continued)

Drug	Common or trade name	Immediate effects	Harmful long-term effects (risk)	Withdrawal effects	Legal status	Use and appeal
STIMULANTS (Continued)						
Cocaine	'Coke'	Local anaesthetic, euphoria, increased energy and alertness. (1)	Restlessness, insomnia, psychosis, suspiciousness, delusions; nausea, digestive disorders, convulsions, ulceration and perforation of the nasal septum. (1)	Psychological dependence. No characteristic physical withdrawal symptoms although depression and delusion may persist for some time. Also prolonged sleepiness. (1)	Illegal for non-medical purposes. Prescription only.	Fashionable recreational use amongst some well-to-do persons. Used because of its euphoric effect and alleged aphrodisiac qualities.
DEPRESSANTS *Alcohol*						
Ethanol	As in wine, spirits, beer, some medicines and household products	Emotional swings, relaxation; impaired judgment, co-ordination, memory and concentration. (1)	Brain, heart, liver, gastric disorders; anaemia, malnutrition; severe mental disorders. (1)	Severe physical and psychological dependence; fitting, vomiting, hallucinations, sweating, delirium tremens. (1)	Illegal for under 18 years and for driving over a prescribed limit.	Generally socially approved. Often segregated use, particularly amongst some social classes. Used as a disinhibitor, social facilitator.

EFFECTS AND EXTENT OF DRUG USE 67

Minor tranquillisers

Oxazepam	Serepax	Reduces anxiety, relaxes muscles, impairs mental and physical abilities. Depression. (5)	Physiological and psychological dependence, vomiting, sweating, nervousness, insomnia, amnesia. (2)	Legal, prescription only.	Widely used to relieve anxiety, especially amongst women.
Diazepam	Valium				
Flunitrazepam	Rohypnol		Depression, fear of withdrawal. (2)		
Chlordiazepoxide	Librium				
Nitrazepam	Mogadon				
Methaqualone	Mandrax (Mandies)	Drowsiness, dizziness. (2)	Psychological, physiological dependence. (2)	Illegal.	In some cases used with alcohol to change effect.

Other prescribed drugs

Amitriptyline HCL	Tryptanol	Cardiac disturbances, drop in blood pressure, light headedness, dry mouth, blurred vision. May be a deterioration in performance. (5)	Possible liver, heart and kidney damage. (5)	Legal, prescription only.	Possible nausea, headaches and malaise on abrupt cessation of amitriptyline. (7)
Doxepin	Sinequan				

Table 8 (continued)

DEPRESSANTS (Continued)

Barbiturates

Drug	Common or trade name	Immediate effects	Harmful long-term effects (risk)	Withdrawal effects	Legal status	Use and appeal
Quinalbarbitone	Seconal	Mild sedative to very intoxicating; forgetfulness, impaired judgment, slurred speech, staggering gait, restlessness, excitement may occur in elderly, coma. (1)	Social dysfunction, dizziness, memory lapses, sleep disturbances, disorientation, allergic reaction, fear of convulsions. (1)	Severe physiological dependence, severe to fatal convulsions, confusion, agitation, delirium, hallucinations, nausea, vomiting, tremor, muscle weakness. (1)	Legal, prescription only.	Any benefits are outweighed by its disadvantages. Other drugs serve same purpose with less negative side effects. Low appeal, some popularity as an intoxicant; cheap and available (although less so than tranquillisers).
Pentobarbitone	Nembutal					
Amylobarbitone	Amytal 'Downers'					

EFFECTS AND EXTENT OF DRUG USE

Narcotics

Drug	Brand	Effects	Risks	Legal status	Extent of use
Heroin	Heroin	Pain relief, euphoria, mood changes, mental clouding, warm flushes, nausea, possible eye pupil changes, depressed respiration. (1)	(Less risk with controlled medical use.) Severe risks of physical disorders (kidney, liver, brain, respiratory, heart, bone, muscles) and infectious diseases (AIDS, skin) from non-medical use. Overdose fatalities. (1)	Heroin illegal. Others legal, prescription only. Prescriber must obtain State Health Authority permission to prescribe for longer than two months. Some used legally for medical purposes.	Illegally used mainly by certain subgroups of late adolescents and young adults, across all social classes. Present trend is difficult to assess.
Morphine	Morphine				
Methadone	Physeptone				
Pethidine	Pethidine		Severe physiological and psychological dependence from chronic use; yawning, muscle tremors, headaches, weakness, sweating, irritability, disturbed sleep, nausea, vomiting, loss of weight, diarrhoea, bone pain, cramps, increased cardiac and respiratory rate. (1)		
Dextromoramide	Palfium				
Hydromorphone	Dilaudid				
Dihydrocodeine	Paracodin				
Propoxyphene	Doloxene				
Buprenorphine	Temgesic				
Codeine	Codeine				
Paracetamol (Acetaminophen)	Panadol	Pain relief, liver failure at high doses. (5)	Liver failure at high doses. (5)	Legal. OTC.	Adult abuse most common amongst lower socio-economic classes. Increasing use amongst adolescents. Appeal provided by analgesia, cheapness and availability.
Aspirin	Vincents	Pain relief, stomach irritation, haemorrhage, anaemia, hearing disturbances. (5)	Stomach and intestinal diseases, haemorrhage, anaemia, hearing disturbances. (5)	Legal. OTC.	
	Aspro		None.		
	Aspirin		None.		

70 OUR DAILY FIX

Table 8 (continued)

Drug	Common or trade name	Immediate effects	Harmful long-term effects (risk)	Withdrawal effects	Legal status	Use and appeal
OTHERS						
Cannabis	Marijuana, Hashish, Bhang, Grass, Hemp	Euphoria, sleepiness; short-term memory, mental and motor skills impairment; senses enhanced, possible hallucinations, delusions, anxiety, increased heart rate. (2)	Respiratory disorders. Impaired judgment, concentration and memory. Loss of energy and motivation have been suggested but evidence is inconclusive. (2)	Physiological dependence has been proposed but not demonstrated. Some appear to be psychologically dependent. (1)	Illegal.	Popularity increasing amongst adolescents. Appeal due to its euphoric and disinhibiting effects and from the thrill of bucking the system.
Chloral hydrate	Noctec	Drowsiness, side effects may include gastric irritation, excitements, confusion, staggering gait, cardiac disturbance. (1)	Possible stomach, kidney and liver damage. Cardiac disturbances. (1)	Physiological dependence. (1)	Legal. Prescription only. Small quantities of dilute solution available OTC in pharmacies in most States.	Particularly by polydrug users, though less popular than in the past. Appealing in its intoxicating effects and cheapness.

EFFECTS AND EXTENT OF DRUG USE 71

Inhalants and solvents (volatile substances)	As in many medical, industrial and common household products	Depends on the substance but may include hyperactivity, excitement, amnesia, exhilaration, impulsiveness, dizziness, nausea, disorientation, hallucinations, drowsiness, stupor, unconsciousness, cardiac arrest. (6)	May include pallor, fatigue, mental impairment, tremors, weight loss, depression, irritability, hostility, feelings of persecution; brain, heart, liver, kidney, blood and nerve damage. (6)	Any dependence would appear to be pyschological. (6)	Legal with warning statements.	Increasing level of use amongst early adolescents. Petrol sniffing prevalent among young Aborigines. Popular because of their availability, cheapness and intoxicating effects.

Note: Use of any of these drugs can cause allergic reactions and/or death.
Sources:
(1) Martindale
(2) Goodman and Gilman
(3) Cox, Jacobs, Leblanc et al.
(4) Avery
(5) Australia, Department of Health, *Australian National Drug Information Service profiles*
(6) Australia, Department of Health, Drugs of Dependence Branch (1984), *Abuse of volatile substances*
(7) Trelearen and Thomas

Extent of drug use in Australia

If you ask most Australians what is the 'drug problem', they will immediately talk about youth, heroin and marijuana. A quick glance at newspaper headlines (such as in Figures 4, 6 and 10) over recent years confirms this impression, and the imagery is heavy with illegality, dirty needles, prostitution, shady deals and drop-out youngsters.

This type of bias confirms our previous propositions about the totems and taboos of drug use. The totem for our society is an ideal, smooth functioning system and anybody deviating from its norms is considered to belong to an aberrant minority whose existence has to be ignored or swept under the mat for fear that it will reflect badly on the ideal. The idea of a taboo is well illustrated by the way in which the reasons for drug abuse, the type of people and substances involved and the extent that society profits from the production and sale of drugs are ignored, glossed over or denied. It is reflected too, in the grudging and limited provision of treatment services, the lack of attention paid to prevention and the removal of many drug problems into the realms of control and imprisonment.

To tell the real story, we examine information which has been provided by the statistics for hospital admissions, mortality, morbidity, accidents, prescriptions, drug sales and consumption, and crime rates. We attempt, as far as possible, to demonstrate which drugs are the real causes of concern. Unfortunately, the amount of reliable, comparable and comprehensive statistics is limited. This is particularly so in regard to the production and use of illegal drugs, because of the nature of the activity. There is also some misreporting of consumption levels of legal drugs such as alcohol and tobacco and among surveys of adolescents. However, the available information on drug use and abuse does go some of the way to correcting the commonly held belief that it is the 'heavy', illegal drugs which cause the most damage.

The following description categorises drugs of concern into three groups, according to, and in order of, the extent of their undesirable impact on health and society, and the numbers of people involved: socially approved recreational drugs, legally prescribed drugs and socially disapproved recreational drugs. The Commonwealth Department of Health (1985) publication, *Statistics on drug abuse in Australia*, prepared for the Special

Premiers' Conference on Drugs, is the source of all the following tables and statistics.

Socially approved recreational drugs (alcohol, nicotine and caffeine)

Without a doubt, alcohol and nicotine are the most commonly used and abused drugs in Australia and have been so for many years. Despite the recent decrease in the numbers of adults who smoke and in the number of road traffic deaths related to alcohol, these substances are still associated with more chronic illnesses, disease, days off work, accidents and personal, family and social problems than all other drugs put together. In Tables 9 and 10, mortality and morbidity figures confirm these propositions.

Some 80 per cent of adult Australians use alcohol although the proportion of regular drinkers has been declining in recent years. However, about 10 per cent of persons aged 25-64 years are regarded to be at risk because they regularly consume over five drinks a day. This is reflected in Table 11 which also shows that men are still heavier users than women, and younger adults drink more heavily but less frequently than older age groups.

Table 9
Admissions to hospitals with a principal diagnosis specifying drug involvement 1981

Drug type	NSW	Qld	WA
Alcohol	13 980	3 619	2 976
Tobacco	6	2	2
Opiates	622	73	47
Cannabis and other hallucinogens	74	26	4
Other drugs	645	313	114
Drug not specified	1 482	255	111
Total drug admissions	16 809	4 288	3 254
Total as % of all admissions	1.6	0.9	1.1

Note: NSW, Qld and WA are the only States with comprehensive hospital morbidity collections covering public and private hospitals.
Source: State Health Authorities

Table 10

Death rates and drugs 1974-83
Deaths per 100 000 population

Drug involved	1974	1975	1976	1977	1978	1979	1980	1981	1982	1983
Alcohol	26.7	26.6	25.8	27.0	26.4	24.6	24.3	23.0	23.6	20.8
Tobacco	121.7	114.4	119.6	113.9	113.4	108.8	110.0	107.9	111.4	108.1
Other drugs										
Opiates	0.6	0.4	0.3	0.4	0.7	0.8	0.6	0.9	1.0	1.3
Barbiturates	0.2	0.3	0.4	0.3	0.3	2.4	1.9	1.3	1.1	0.9
Other	5.6	5.3	4.6	4.6	5.1	2.2	2.1	1.7	2.0	2.5
Total	6.4	6.0	5.3	5.4	6.1	5.4	4.6	4.0	4.1	4.7
Total, all drugs	154.8	147.1	150.7	146.3	145.9	138.8	138.9	134.9	139.1	133.6

Note: Prior to 1979 some deaths due to opiate or barbiturate use are included in 'Other' under 'Other drugs'

Table 11
Drinking patterns among persons aged 25-64 years, Australian State capital cities, 1980 and 1983
(per cent)

	Males				Females			
	25-34 years		35-64 years		25-34 years		35-64 years	
Drinking pattern	1980	1983	1980	1983	1980	1983	1980	1983
Frequency of drinking								
Non-drinkers	5	9	11	13	13	18	22	28
Occasional drinkers[a]	71	75	52	55	75	74	59	56
Regular drinkers[b]	24	16	37	32	12	8	20	16
Amount usually consumed on a drinking day								
1-4 drinks	67	73	74	80	93	92	96	96
5-8 drinks	26	19	18	15	6	7	4	4
9 or more drinks	7	7	8	5	1	0	0	0
Use of low alcohol beer by beer drinkers[c]								
None or small proportion	73	72	75	67	74	70	75	67
About half of all beer	9	13	8	12	5	9	5	6
Most or all of beer	18	15	18	22	21	21	20	28
Distribution of risk levels								
Non-drinkers or low risk	89	93	85	89	95	96	93	93
Intermediate risk	9	6	10	8	5	3	6	6
High and very high risk	3	2	5	2	1	1	1	1

a Up to four days per week
b Five or more days per week
c Proportion of beer drunk as low alcohol beer
Source: National Heart Foundation of Australia, p. 8

Although the overall number of smokers has fallen slightly in recent years, the figures for the age group with the greatest prevalence of smoking (25-34 years) have remained stable at 36 per cent for men and 28 per cent for women. Table 12 illustrates the extent of use amongst the various age groups and the proportion of smokers, ex-smokers and non-smokers. All smokers are at risk from tobacco-related illnesses while ex-smokers (50 per cent of men and 32 per cent of women) have a reduced risk.

The one group where use of both alcohol and nicotine has increased quite dramatically is the young, as is shown in Table 13. Alcohol consumption has reportedly more than doubled while tobacco use, which was more prevalent in 1971, has also increased but only slightly. Table 13 shows that both substances are used more regularly by high school students than any other type of drug.

Caffeine is included in this section not because of its lethal effects but because it is so widely used, because it can be abused and because it has chronic effects which may be of some significance. It is possibly the most underrated drug in common use. Moderate use does not appear to be harmful but there are large individual differences in susceptibility. An excessive dose is regarded as chronic use of over seven cups of instant coffee a day (or the equivalent in tea, chocolate or cola drinks). However, children, who have a lower body weight, can fall into the at risk category with, for example, only three cokes and three chocolate bars in a day.

Gilliland and Bullock regard caffeine as a potential drug of abuse because an estimated 10-20 per cent of Americans are at risk from 'Caffeinism', the effects of which include withdrawal symptoms, chronic depression, anxiety, irritability, headaches and altered work performance. Because caffeine is not generally considered as a drug, such symptoms may not be recognised as being due to its use. No figures are available on the incidence of 'Caffeinism' in Australia but the research information suggests that this is an area which needs to be better understood.

Legal medications (pain relievers, stimulants, depressants)
Drugs are prescribed in the normal course of health care, for pain, depression, anxiety, stress, and the disorientation of the elderly. In regard to the number of people involved, their impact on health and their implications for problem-solving behaviour, the misuse

Table 12

Smoking patterns among persons aged 25-64 years, Australian State capital cities, 1980 and 1983

Smoking pattern		Males				Females			
		25-34 years		35-64 years		25-34 years		35-64 years	
		1980	1983	1980	1983	1980	1983	1980	1983
Cigarette smoker [a,b]	%	36	36	35	30	28	28	25	24
Cigar and/or pipe only	%	3	1	4	3				
Ex-smoker	%	20	20	30	32	15	16	15	16
Never smoked regularly	%	40	43	31	35	57	56	60	61
Cigarettes per day [c]	(No.)	18	20	23	22	16	14	15	17
21 plus cigarettes daily [d]	%	34	33	47	44	27	16	21	24

a May also smoke cigars or pipe
b Includes manufactured and 'hand-rolled' cigarettes
c Average number of manufactured cigarettes smoked daily
d Proportion of cigarette smokers who smoke 21 or more manufactured cigarettes daily

Source: National Heart Foundation of Australia, p. 9

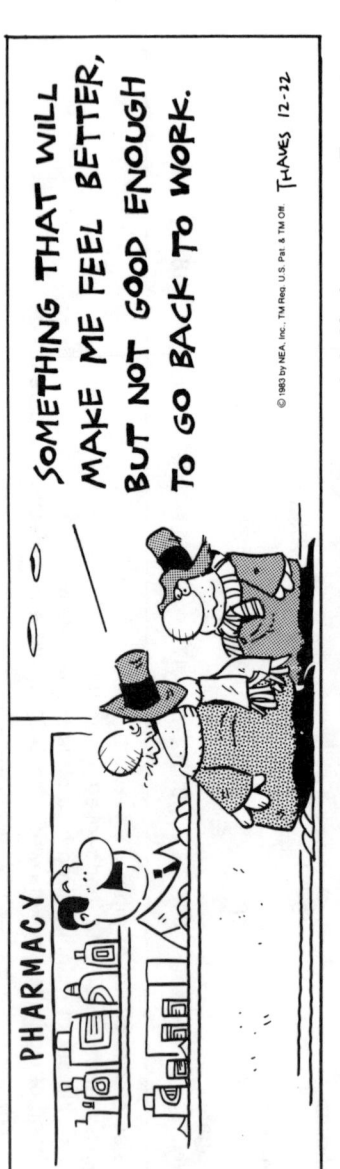

Cartoon by Thaves, reprinted by permission of United Press International on behalf of Newspaper Enterprise Association, from *Australian*, 19 December 1983

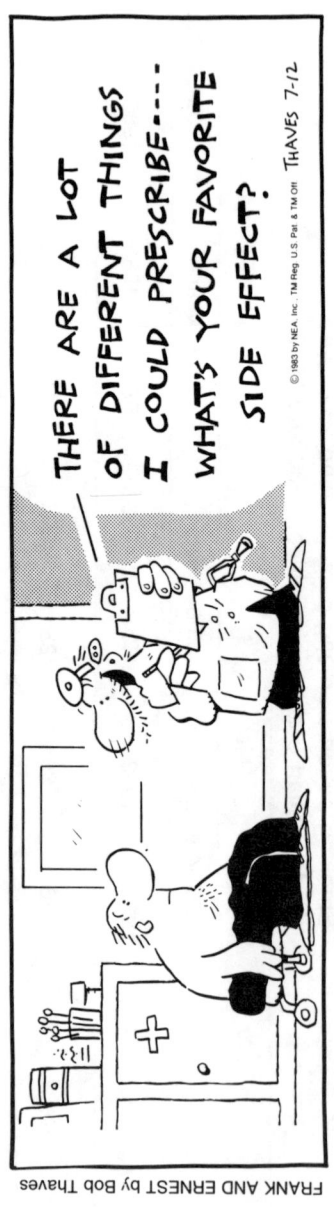

Cartoon by Thaves, reprinted by permission of United Press International on behalf of Newspaper Enterprise Association, from *Australian*, 8 March 1984

Table 13

Weekly drug use by year 10 students,
New South Wales, 1971-83 (per cent)

Drug type	1971	1973	1977	1980	1983
	N = 3300	N = 3369	N = 492	N = 395	N = 755
Alcohol	22	31	38	33	50
Tobacco	29	30	40	35	35
Analgesics	16	15	11	21	30
Cannabis (marijuana)	2	4	8	6	12
Sedatives	4	4	3	3	2
Hallucinogens	1	1	1	1	2
Stimulants	4	3	2		2
Narcotics			1	1	

Source: New South Wales Drug and Alcohol Authority

and abuse of legal medications rates as the second most important area of concern. There is a huge range of prescription and over the counter drugs which serve very useful purposes, if used as directed. However, the basic instructions which accompany each product are frequently misunderstood or ignored. The significance of that important advice is often unappreciated, sometimes in ignorance, sometimes on purpose.

The situation reflects a very casual and naive attitude to the nature of drugs and suggests a socially approved basis for drug use in all sections of society. These sections include the legislators who allow potentially dangerous products to be, in many cases, freely available to all ages; the doctors who prescribe drugs rather than take time to consider alternatives; pharmacists who dispense without discussion; advertisers who plug their products as risk free, cure-alls; parents who medicate their children at the mere sign of a problem; and people generally, who regard drugs as the quick, easy way to fix all problems without having to make much effort, let alone confront the reasons. Common sweets are dispensed from 'pill' type packages; aspirin are packed in children's lunch boxes. The prescribed drug as 'totem' of health and well-being is strongly integrated into our daily lives.

Misuse is one part of the problem. It is apparently widespread throughout all age groups, with people taking the wrong drug for the wrong reason, taking the wrong dose ('if one is good, two must be better') and taking drugs unnecessarily.

Non-compliance and abuse are of particular concern also, particularly in the way they result in the unnecessary filling of hospital beds with patients who overdose, who have had inappropriate therapy, who have had adverse reactions or who have become dependent on a drug. Reasons include deliberate risk taking, lack of explanation from doctors, lack of explanation from the pharmacist, unclear labelling, inadequate questioning and understanding by the patient and, most of all, general ignorance by the user about the properties of drugs especially in regard to dosage, side effects and mixing different types.

The extent of current use of prescription items alone is clearly demonstrated by the large numbers of scripts written and the enormous amount of money spent on them. In 1983-84, according to the Annual Report of the Commonwealth Department of Health 109 000 scripts were written valued at $649 million.

The 1983 Australian Health Survey indicated wide usage when it reported that 47 per cent of people, including children, had taken some form of legal drug in the two days preceding the interview (see Table 14).

The most commonly used drugs were the pain relievers and the preliminary figures for 1984 suggest their use (at least for prescription items) is increasing, unlike other substances (except vitamins and minerals). Further evidence of the popularity of pain relievers is shown by the figures from the New South Wales Drug and Alcohol Authority survey of year 10 habits which showed that the percentage using them had doubled to 30 over the past decade (see Table 13).

Reports of poison cases admitted to hospitals also give reasons for concern about legal medications. Benzodiazepines such as Valium were the drugs most commonly involved, accounting for 26 per cent of all cases, while pain relievers accounted for 9 per cent and antidepressants for 6 per cent. (Alcohol accounted for 11 per cent and opiates for 2 per cent.)

Another reflection on the extent of abuse of legal medications is shown by the fact that the incidence of serious renal disease in Australia is still significantly higher than in other countries and

Table 14
Australian Health Surveys 1977-78 and 1983:
persons taking medication in the two days before interview
(percentage of population in same age group)

Type of medication	0-14 years		15-34 years		35 years +		All ages	
	1977-78	1983	1977-78	1983	1977-78	1983	1977-78	1983
Pain relievers	8	6	15	11	21	19	16	13
Cough medicine	9	7	4	3	5	3	6	4
Allergy medicine	2	2	3	3	3	3	3	3
Tranquillisers	1	1	2	1	9	6	5	3
Sleeping pills			1	1	6	6	3	3
Vitamins, minerals	12	18	11	21	11	23	12	21

Source: Australian Bureau of Statistics

reflects a serious analgesic abuse problem among certain sections of the population, particularly lower socio-economic groups and Aborigines. The rate per million has increased in persons aged 50-69 years in New South Wales from ten people in 1972 to forty-five in 1983.

The measures which have been introduced to reduce compound analgesic use have as yet had no perceptible impact on the numbers involved. It is suspected that this situation may be due to the long lead time required to develop the disorder or that new use patterns are equally as damaging as those that were suppressed. Table 15 reveals that use is rising rather than falling.

Although there are no figures available, the Pharmaceutical Society of Australia suspects that there may be something in the order of 30 000 people who chronically misuse over the counter preparations.

Comparatively less of a problem but still also of concern are the illegal use of forged prescriptions and the obtaining of drugs under false pretences—however there are few figures to demonstrate the extent of these problems.

The use of drugs in sport is another cause for concern and it is believed that the level of misuse in this area is increasing, for instance, the use of sympathomimetics by swimmers and caffeine by cyclists. Although large numbers are not involved, the extent of the influence of sporting champions on the young must increase our anxiety at the trend.

Socially disapproved recreational drugs (narcotics, cocaine, hallucinogens, cannabis, volatile substances).

Even though the numbers of those affected by abuse of these substances is small in comparison with the previously mentioned drugs, the following substances rate as significant because of their effect on health and social functioning, because their use involves illegal behaviour and because of their attraction for the young.

Narcotics: Although few people are willing to put figures on the extent of use (and any such figures would have to be guesstimates), the generally held view is that it is increasing, especially among the young. Deaths from narcotics in the figures from the Sydney Coroner's Court (Table 16) show that although the years of life lost are considerable because of the youth of victims, the actual numbers involved are few. In 1974 there were four deaths, in 1979 they had risen to thirty-eight and in 1980 there were twenty-two.

Table 15

Prescriptions for psychopharmaceuticals and total prescriptions under the Pharmaceutical Benefits Scheme 1974-75 to 1983-84 (prescriptions per 100 000 population)

Drug group	1975	1976	1977	1978	1979	1980	1981	1982	1983	1984p
Analgesics	680	732	696	787	793	806	825	811	854	921
Major tranquillisers	70	70	65	60	59	56	54	55	53	52
Minor tranquillisers (Valium and Serepax)	378	342	246	262	239	200	195	273	238	210
Anti-depressants	248	261	239	247	236	226	224	233	231	233
Hypnotics and sedatives	334	300	210	242	198	185	171	179	183	180
Other drug groups	5359	5535	4901	4926	4902	4678	4926	5331	5351	5462
Total	7069	7240	6358	6524	6427	6151	6394	6883	6910	7058

p = preliminary

Table 16
Deaths[a] involving drugs reported upon by Sydney Coroner's Court 1972-80 (number)

Drug involved	1972	1973	1974	1975	1976	1977	1978	1979	1980
Barbiturates	146	143	112	129	125	98	88	144	110
Alcohol	98	110	93	141	131	127	111	75	81
Narcotics	8	7	4	10	25	33	32	38	22
Other	73	49	70	80	47	42	38	44	36

a: Excludes deaths from traffic accidents

Cocaine: Cocaine is currently fashionable and its use is believed to be increasing but still low in comparison with other illegal drugs.

Hallucinogens: Hallucinogens have periodic bursts of popularity during which they are widely used by certain social subgroups. According to the New South Wales study their use by students in year 10 is very low compared to other drugs.

Cannabis: Cannabis is the fourth most widely used drug among youth, after alcohol, tobacco and analgesics, and its use appears to be increasing. The New South Wales survey indicated that in 1983 12 per cent used it regularly. It is believed that some 3-5 per cent of adults also use it regularly.

Volatile substances: The area of volatile substances is one of the most difficult to describe because it is associated with a great variety of easily available substances, many of which are common in households and work places. They are of concern particularly because of their attraction to children who use them experimentally (although older people are involved with the use of some substances) and because some can cause instant death.

There are few data on the use of volatile substances and what information there is may be unreliable. The 1983 survey of New South Wales secondary schools indicated that the sniffing of solvents and aerosols was most common among early adolescents, with 50 per cent reporting that they had sniffed at least once. One per cent reported sniffing every day. There did not appear to be any discernible pattern amongst users in regard to their social class, type of school or location. The level of use was higher than reported in USA.

Conclusion

The picture painted by these facts and figures is that Australia is a country in which a daily 'quick fix' is a normal part of most people's lives. Use is firmly established in childhood with the types of drugs being used varying over the life cycle (see Table 5). The other feature of these data is that legal status has little to do with the severity of a drug's effects and merely labels a drug 'good' or 'bad' in a way which camouflages its real impact on health and welfare. Ignorance and desperation appear to be the main reasons for misuse and abuse. Risk taking accounts for experimental use by the young groups, which they will grow out of, if they survive.

Ignorance, desperation and risk taking are all individual states, dependent on the encompassing society. What it is to be ignorant differs from place to place. Eskimos have twenty-four words for snow; our children spend eleven years at school without necessarily learning how their own bodies work, or their own society functions; both human biology and civics are optional units in most schools. With the added confusion of technical terms for familiar physical functions, is it any wonder that the 'one dose and you are hooked' mythology persists in the community, against medical and streetwise knowledge. It is not only the drug takers who are ignorant. How to put our high degree of biochemical, psychological and physiological knowledge to work in reducing drug abuse is a central question, which we must try to answer.

PART 2

STRATEGIES:
Reducing Drug Abuse

5
Our Heads In The World

Translating will to deed

Part 1 has dealt with the world of ideas, that is, the formulation of policy, its importance and the effects it has on attitudes to drug abuse. To stop there would leave us with our heads in the clouds: the next step is to put those heads into the world. A balanced understanding of what can be called 'the facts' has been the object of the exercise so far; now we need to understand decisions to act. Hence, we review the various strategies used in dealing with drug abuse, namely Control, Treatment, Education and Social Change, in the light of the social context, the extent of drug use, and the present directions of policy.

Schein has noted that effective action requires two separate phases: a desire for the action by those in charge of policy, and acceptance by those who actually have to carry out the program. But the transition from ideas to action is not quite so simple. There is a vital middle step, often ignored, with which we all, policy maker, strategist and program deliverer, have to deal.

Policy and social rules are the expressions of public norms. The totems and taboos involved are therefore highly visible and very powerful, but it is not the 'public' which has to act on that policy: it is actual individuals. Therefore the policy will only succeed if those individuals genuinely accept and understand that policy for themselves, and if their own private totems are consistent with the action. Real understanding requires some translation of an abstract policy into tangible terms, related to the environment of the translator. For example, it is all very well to have a policy calling for a 'neighbourhood watch' scheme to report drug traffickers to the police. That will not succeed until the people in the suburb see the need for such a scheme—and that understanding requires a translation of the problem on a personal level. It is one thing to talk about 4000 drug addicts. It is quite another to find syringes on your front lawn or in your son's bedroom.

As a tool of translation from ideas to action, we need a common understanding of the nature and extent of the problem; a common view of the real world of drug abuse, the statistics and the physiological effects of use and the results of abuse. We need to understand the links between thought and performance for all those charged with acting on drug abuse.

It is often thought that the role of understanding facts and determining strategies is the function of the professional. Surely the purpose of their training is not merely to develop ideas but to put them into practice? But it is not enough just to accept that lawyer or doctor knows best. This is especially so the more comprehensive the avenue of approach or response that is favoured. Control, perhaps, can be imposed without understanding in the community or by other professions, but it will be far more effective with it. For instance, random breath testing has received remarkable public support, support based on agreement with the policy and understanding the effectiveness of the strategy. Effective treatment is more and more being recognised as depending on the understanding, co-operation, and participation of the patient or client. Ironically, tests showing the efficacy of placebos go some way to demonstrate this, and it is a fundamental tenet of many of the branches of alternative medicine. Education will not succeed in the development of acceptable social norms without the implicit consent of parents as well as teachers. And social change, by its very nature, demands understanding, knowledge and support from all of the community. The world of ideas has such an all-pervading effect on attitudes to drugs that it would be easy to leave it there, as a communication problem. But once abuse is the issue, we have the paradox of taboos and totems reversed, and our game of tic-tac-totem is back. If heroin is illegal, and taboo, how can we rehabilitate the abusers? Officially they don't exist. Just as policy makes no sense without the social context from which it grew, so strategies are inseparable from the information on which they are based. Information that methadone now has a 'street' use as a drug of abuse has confused the professional use of methadone as a replacement strategy in heroin treatment.

Facts

What is being discussed here is factual, but what is 'a fact' must be kept in perspective. The phrase 'objective facts' is often bandied about as some sort of totem of our faith in a world ultimately determinable by scientists. But the phrase is not a tautology, rather it is a contradiction in terms. Facts are not absolutes of truth, they are a collection of different types of values. Facts are first gathered, and then interpreted in the light of subjective beliefs and experiences which colour them and give them meaning. Although this is true of scientific information in general (for instance, the nuclear debate), potential conflict between fact and value reaches its height in the area of drugs. From research workers who decide what to investigate to field workers who must act on the findings there is seldom an uninterrupted straight line along which logical argument can flow.

Facts must, by definition, have both objective and subjective elements. They are needed for the translation of abstract policy into action, but they themselves are the result of a choice of action, and require interpretation before they are of use. Of what meaning is the information that there are 4000 heroin addicts in Australia —or 40 000, or 400 000—unless we impose on that the image of what is a tolerable level? To do that we must know what these people look like, what they are forgoing by being addicted, our own view of the value of human potential, and so on. And how can that fact stimulate action or reaction, in contrast to the claims of outrage and concern at the fact that, say, 3000 people die every year in road deaths, until we impose a complex series of beliefs based on the morality of drugs, or the worth to our economy of efficient road transport, or the fact that it is our son or daughter who is addicted or was run over by a drunken driver? The politician and the professional are not absolved from this level, whatever the myth of the objective observer. Queensland's health care system is strongly influenced by a Premier saved from crippling poliomyelitis by (at that time) unorthodox treatment. Two of the more successful rehabilitation units are reflections of the experiences of ex-addicts. Do we value risk taking in our young so highly that we supply the right to drink alcohol, economic independence, and access to potentially lethal substances in the same year of their lives?

Facts are based on values, and values sneak in regardless, including those of the authors. For example, in Chapter 6, it is said of cannabis that it is 'probably no worse than alcohol or tobacco', and this is physiologically accurate. It implies, however, a judgment derived from our social concern with the effects of these products, and a downgrading of certain sociological arguments, which is based on the values and priorities of the authors. We apologise, but since we regard a value position as inevitable, we ask you to look carefully at the world in your own head and not to expect us to set ours aside.

Evidence

It is this overlay of values which creates evidence—for evidence is collected for a *purpose*; to prove something, or as the basis of some theory or belief. These values are the sieve through which empirical evidence is filtered by the observer. But this sieve is itself made up of facts of various sorts which can be tested and examined: ethical values, based on the moral, political, religious and personal beliefs of the community; aesthetic values drawn from the culture of our society, what it appreciates or what it considers good or beautiful, bad or ugly; and social values created by the political and legal rules of the society and the way it creates role stereotypes. Moreover, this sieving process is infinite. Facts are put through this value-sieve by the observer, but the very choice of what facts to observe is based on his/her values, and on conclusions from past experienceswhich are themselves the result of this value process, and so on. The present epidemic of over-medication of the ageing has its roots in a generation able to accept the promise of a pharmaceutical cure, having been adults through the 'miracle' of antibiotics as cures, and before the lifestyle diseases needing behaviour change as cures.

The point of all this is not just to allow the reader to be aware of the complex value processes involved in interpreting facts. As far as the reader is concerned, these facts are already second or third hand. They have already gone through several processes. Therefore, to interpret and evaluate them properly requires careful consideration of more than the empirical data. The whole is demonstrably greater than the sum of the parts and a more holistic approach is required to properly act on the reports of a scientific problem or a social situation. In considering, let us say, the abuse of anabolic steroids by sports people, it is necessary to consider not only the statistical data on that abuse, but the ethical position that encourages athletic excellence and winning, the aesthetic that admires natural beauty over that which is artificially enhanced, the intricate set of rules which govern sports, as well as the aims and goals of the sports person herself and how all these factors have influenced the observer.

These considerations are vital in evaluating the strategies discussed here. Consider a proposal for harsher penalties for the abuse of prescribed drugs. Behind this lies the complex sieve of assumptions through which evidence has been filtered in order to conclude that such a measure is necessary. There are the *ethical* or moral values that dictate that society has a right to control self-willed actions by autonomous members, and that punishment is an effective deterrent. The *aesthetic* values are often overlooked, but are powerful determinants of action. Imagine the order and cleanliness of the white pill in a hospital—and the contrast of the untidy room, pills scattered everywhere, a body slumped aslant the bed. And what of the *social* values which put responsibility for prescribing drugs into the hands of doctors, and trust that judgment totally? Medical opinion for nearly a decade was that Valium was not addictive, and had no severe side effects. Wrong on both counts, as our drug tables record. These factors may together demand that control measures be advocated—or they may not. The strategy cannot be evaluated properly without considering all the factors, the world in the head brought to bear upon the head in the world.

Table 17 describes the collection of the necessary evidence to act on a drug issue, the methods available for gathering that evidence, and the appropriate test by which the validity of the evidence can be confirmed: measurement and experiment for physical dimensions of an issue, observation of moral positions for the ethical dimension, standards of taste for the aesthetic influences, rules of behaviour for the social component, finally range of individual perspectives which contribute to the whole pattern of response.

We can now apply the evidence collected on all five aspects of an issue to any drug problem we wish to consider. For an example, we can examine the use and abuse of heroin (Table 18) in the light of the framework for drug issues developed in Tables 2 and 7, and with respect to the various aspects of evidence. Consideration of the physical aspects gives us a baseline for what is achievable in control and treatment, etc.; of the ethical aspects gives us what is

Table 17
Choosing a strategy : collecting the evidence

Aspects of evidence	Collected by	Validated by
Physical states	Observation, measurement, experiment	Repetition, reproducibility, probability, prediction
Ethical goals	Observation of behaviour, reports of intentions, and moral positions	Consistency, reliability; reflected in myths, symbols, and rituals
Aesthetic responses	Observation of behaviour, artefacts, statements of taste and feeling	Relationship to standards, of taste and beauty, reliability, sincerity
Social rules	Observation of behaviour, norms, roles and institutions	Consensus, reliability, acceptability
Individual perspectives	Self-report of moral position, standards of taste and feeling, norms, rules and roles	Reliability, internal consistency, sincerity and introspection

Table 18
Framework for drug issues 4: strategy analysis—responses to heroin use

Aspects of the issue	Avenues of approach			
	Control	Treatment	Education	Social change
Physical states (impact of action)	Methadone replaces heroin addiction	See Figure 13 for effects; not necessarily addictive; addiction treatable	Pharmacology and physiology very well known; not usually taught	Users often pass unnoticed; abusers show severe physical impairment
Ethical goals (policy)	Taboo: all heroin use is a sin and a crime	Heroin use is an illness, and so must be treated	Use and abuse are from ignorance	Heroin users beginning to be seen as victims of society
Aesthetic responses (social context)	Ugly and repulsive habits	Messy, unclean and destructive of the person	Rituals of use reinforce addiction	Escape from harsh reality for some; a sense of belonging for others
Social rules (social content)	Criminal empires founded on heroin supply; police tempted, laws inadequate	Contact with addicts is polluting for (pure) health care providers	Heroin is taboo, therefore cannot be mentioned in formal education	Heroin is taboo for law abiders; totem for law breakers
Individual perspective (the actors—here, an ordinary citizen)	Control keeps me safe from law breakers	Treatment keeps me and mine safe from contagion	I need to know more; if users knew more, they wouldn't use it	More citizens accepting that abuse is widespread; sometimes their own children

acceptable, and of the social aspects, what is permissible. We can consider what an ordinary citizen, a lawyer or an addict might consider the position to be, and so gradually build up a three-dimensional picture of the whole.

6
Control

Catch 22

Control can be exercised over drug users not merely by the imposition of legal regulation, but in the aim and exercise of treatment methods, in the education of school students and of course by the power of strongly held social values. Indeed, why are we concerned with drug abuse at all? It is not simply because of our concern for the state of health of the citizens. Earle Hackett says in the Postscript that drug abuse threatens 'attitudes to neurochemical by-passing of the human motivation to work' and the social desire for conformity. Social desires are often to 'solve the drug problem' as a means of controlling the behaviour of members and keeping their rebellion, eccentricity and expressions of individuality within limits. The law is a very powerful totem, and is invoked to see that other social symbols, such as work, family, government and commerce, are not infringed.

The most obvious way in which the social control is manifested is by the imposition of laws and penalties aimed at the punishment, restriction and deterrence of drugs and users. The strategies which perhaps receive more publicity than any other are those directed towards the legal control of drugs and drug users. Questions such as the legal availability of cannabis and methadone, enforced treatment of addicts, stiffer penalties and greater police powers have received a great deal of airplay, news space and public comment.

This is intensified by the limited contribution that individual members of a society can make to the long-term minimisation of drug abuse. This is not surprising; laws are, as was mentioned in

Chapter 5, the rules and framework that people construct for society, and although these are often seen as the expression of the ethical values of the society, ethics and laws serve clearly different purposes. Laws are not only considered as the representation of social ethics, they in turn mould them. There is a two-way process in much the same way as there is between policy and social context (see Chapter 3). Thus, the social attitude to alcohol and heroin respectively is reflected in their legal status. But the very status of a drug as illegal defines social attitudes to it. Much of the interest in using cannabis is described by cannabis users as exactly *because* their behaviour is illegal. The breaking of a law is itself seen as a breach of normal social behaviour and a challenge to the existing ethic of the system. Drug use thus acquires a social function for the individual, quite apart from its effects. To bring a taboo into the light of day by breaking it forces a society to recognise the individual and reassess the taboo.

Here is Catch 22.

The very power of the complex interactions between legal rules and social norms makes a critical analysis of laws important. But one of these social norms is that laws should be complied with without undue criticism. It is a strong totem of social cohesion that laws be accepted. There is then a strong monkey-grip for conformity. But although the law may be a codified norm, it is not a constant; but changes with ethical positions.

The law is often unresponsive to change, however, and can ossify the beliefs and needs of a different age. Therefore a questioning approach is vital. In recent years, that we are in an age of social change has been recognised, with more frequent debate on legal issues and the growth in publicity and resources given to the various Federal and State Law Reform Commissions.

In this chapter, it is intended to give a critical perspective on the issues and options that lie in the legal control of drugs. Licit and illicit drugs are treated separately, not because there is any evidential validity in such a distinction from a policy perspective, but because the legal strategies currently implemented are obviously very different in these areas. Illicit drugs are approached with the desire to suppress, and licit drugs with the desire to control. It is vital then, in reading this chapter, to appreciate that just because the law is a certain way this is not necessarily how it should be.

Illicit drugs

International efforts
There is a significant degree of consensus in the world community over drugs. Specifically, there is commonly a condemnation of a number of specific drugs, and a belief in the utility of strict control measures to deal with them. It is less common for governments to recognise the often perfunctory way in which such a consensus is arrived at before being entrenched as 'international law'.

International efforts are over-ambitious, fragmented and supply oriented. Programs such as the encouragement of poor villagers to replace their opium with other cash crops are worthy of Australian support. But as long as world demand for illicit drugs continues, these programs merely shift the centres of drug production. Furthermore, current international efforts centred on supply and control have been largely unsuccessful. Governments in the Golden Triangle of opium/heroin production lack the will, power or resources to effectively restrict the exportation of these goods. It may therefore be useful for Australia to encourage more action centred on demand, treatment and prevention, within the UN system, although research into altering the type of poppy grown for therapeutic purposes is one supply-oriented measure that holds some promise.

International obligations
The Conventions to which Australia is signatory (Convention on Psychotropic Substances and Single Convention on Narcotic Drugs) involve a complex set of measures to control production and supply. Most controversial is the classification of cannabis as a narcotic, subject to 'special measures' due to its 'particularly dangerous properties'. This categorisation is questionable, and many reports and commissions have emphasised the importance of a more realistic classification (for an Australian overview, see Table 1). Whether an attempt by Australia to remedy the situation would meet with international support is arguable. Many countries and international organisations are adamant about maintaining strict controls in this area.

Any relaxation in cannabis laws would be against international law and amity. This is not to say that Australia should necessarily follow international law. However it should be taken into account and, if necessary, means should be devised to justify Australia's position without losing the present measure of international goodwill. Perhaps a greater involvement in international efforts would shore up Australia's reputation in this area.

Legalisation
Legalisation is not an all or nothing affair. It may involve allowing possession of a drug but not sale, or developing a state marketing monopoly, or reducing penalties for possession to a mere fine, like parking offences (decriminalisation), or permitting open trade on certain conditions (restriction on place and time of sale as with alcohol). Proposals to legalise and regulate *all* drugs have been carefully argued for on the basis that the law has failed to suppress drug abuse. It is impossible to tell, however, what the situation would have been without such controls. Civil liberty arguments have also been strongly made on this point, but the present community climate in relation to 'hard drugs' makes any far-reaching control relaxation, even if desirable, difficult to achieve. Support to legalise cannabis has mounted because of the large and growing number of users. This is especially true in USA where a number of States have decriminalised. Legalisation of narcotics would be more acceptable in the face of a dramatic upsurge in users; hardly a situation to be encouraged.

However, controlled legalisation has certain advantages. The main options include legal availability to registered addicts (sometimes called the 'British system'), a state monopoly, or a system of supervised licensed dealers. One of the main harmful consequences of drug use is the property crime committed by users. If, for example, heroin were legally available, or available to addicts, the illicit market would be undercut, and crime and organised crime would be minimised. This argument can be over-emphasised—many addicts rely on employment, not illegal means, to finance their habit. Moreover, a large percentage of addicts have a history of delinquency and crime predating drug use. Therefore the extent to which drug abuse is the major factor in non drug-related crime is questionable.

If drug use is considered a health rather than a social problem, it is a great mistake to think that the drug itself is the prime cause of illness. Problems caused by unsanitary syringe practices, such as AIDS and hepatitis, and by impurities and variances in the street-level drug are the real killers. Changes in legislation which allow a greater level of health care and supervision in a system of at least partial legality may assist. Laws based on illegality and suppression, for example stiffer penalties for selling syringes, could actually increase the level of health risks.

Supply
Many drugs may continue to be controlled by means directed at supply and trafficking. Supply controls are still largely a question of internal steps to restrict entry of illegal drugs into the country, all of which except cannabis are mainly imported. Other countries' efforts to stop exportation have failed. Given this, the Customs barrier is a vital front line. The Customs Act gives considerable powers to search, seize, arrest and penalise, but there are at present no adequate resources to enforce the Act. Customs inspection in Australia is less vigorous than in many other countries, and important ports are insufficiently staffed.

However, the importance of this aspect must be weighed against the many other ways of smuggling drugs into Australia. Northern Australia is a smuggler's dream. A tighter Customs screen may catch many couriers, but is unlikely to inhibit large commercial operations. Heroin importation into Australia has not been highly organised, but Woodward indicated that the market was ripe for

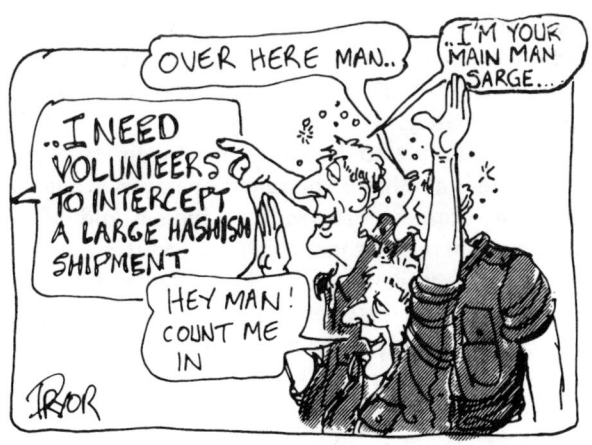

Cartoon by Pryor, reprinted by permission of Pryor of the **Canberra Times**, *from* **Canberra Times**, *26 February 1985*

more central control. Stewart's investigations indicate that that process is under way.

Coastal surveillance in Australia is very disorganised. There are those who argue that a 100 per cent cordon is economically viable, but it would seem to be impossible. More cost-effective means to improve coastal surveillance include a less ad hoc approach to the purchase of new patrol boats and aeroplanes; an analysis of high risk areas, and rationalisation of resources; the retention of manned lighthouses; and the use of meteorological radar.

The use of radar is a promising idea, but the device's detail and accuracy are unproven. A more drastic suggestion is the development of a compulsory non-military National Service which would be involved in coastal surveillance among other things. In the end, the amount spent on upgrading surveillance depends on the extent to which it is believed that supply controls can limit drug use. The willingness of supply sources to take whatever risks are necessary to reap huge profits should not be forgotten.

Trafficking

In recent years there has been a general trend combining sympathy towards users with advocating harsher penalties for traffickers. In a rough way this is valid, but to some extent it is illogical. Indeed, the present trafficking offences are currently wide enough to encompass those who purchase for their own use. Moreover, almost all traffickers are primarily users who sell to support their habit. Those who advocate minimum penalties ignore this. At present, judicial flexibility in sentencing allows punishment to be adjusted appropriately.

Arguments continue to be raised in favour of even tougher penalties. While a number of marginal operators would be forced out of business, those who stayed in business would have a larger, assured, market share and charge higher prices to accommodate the extra risk. The effect would be continued demand, greater profits and a more organised network. In addition, if higher penalties applied to cannabis, dealers would be encouraged to turn to more profitable, concealable drugs like heroin.

The power to confiscate the profits of a crime or the assets of a drug trafficker is not solely for reasons of deterrence. It is also

Figure 6   Heroin in the headlines (at right)

Aussie two in drug test case

GEORGETOWN, Penang — with the trial here today of two Australians on drug trafficking charges, the world will realise Malaysia is serious in its drugs war.

The trial will be a test case of Asian resolve to tackle the drug menace.

The two Australians, Geoff ..., 28, of Perth, and ... ..., 28, of Adelaide, face the prospect of mandatory hanging if convicted

Heroin smuggler collapses in court

A MAN fainted in the County Court yesterday then struggled with police after he was sentenced to jail for heroin importation.

Bahri Kural, 25, was found guilty by a jury of having imported the drug with a street value of more than $520,000.

Kural, formerly of Tatura, was a drug courier arrested at Tullamarine in March 1983.

He had hidden 468 g of heroin in the base of an electric Turkish teapot, which Kural claimed he was given by a stranger at Istanbul to bring to Melbourne.

Judge Ostrowski said: "I have no doubt at all that you knew what you were doing and that you did it for money."

Kural had smarted at being unable to provide for his family because he had an injury.

The tomato picker had been ordered by his father, president of the Turkish community in Goulburn Valley, to leave the area.

Turkish family and friends in the court wept when the judge ordered 10 years jail with a minimum term of a seven years.

As Kural was led from the court he collapsed. Water was poured on him to revive him and he then struggled as he was being taken to the cells.

FROM DRUG ADDICT TO CATS SUPERSTAR

DAILY TELEGRAPH, Saturday, July 6, 1985

Court hears of heroin, killing link

A MAN charged over the importation of heroin valued at nearly $8 million was wanted for questioning over the killing of underworld figure Daniel Chuk... ...was told yesterday.

Allan Goldsworthy alleged ...ed in ...eek to ...ained ...ases in. ...f ...rgeant ...ed Ho... Sydney ho... been und... by police, suitcase deposit...

PICTURE: BRUCE MILLER

Debbie moving triumph

JUST over two years ago a thin and emotionally fragile Debbie Byrne checked out of a Sydney drug rehabilitation centre and began to rebuild her life.

The career of the two... winner and...

KIDNAPPER DUMPED

From DARREN HORRIGAN in Melbourne

THE kidnapper who walked out of jail last week by swapping identities with another prisoner has been found dead, dumped in bushland.

Ian Leslie Sutton, aged 33, a known heroin addict, is believed to have died of a drug overdose.

His fully-clothed body was found late yesterday beside a dirt road outside Bendigo, about 95 km north of Melbourne.

...last week Pentridge ...rities and ...he swapped ...another pri... ...back on their ...out to jail ...while on their ...e man was ...o Pentridge for the non-payment of a $100 fine.

Sutton was going for a ... robberies...

JAIL SWAP MAN 'DIES OF DRUGS'

Police were aware of his escape only after an "outside tip-off".

They have ruled out foul play but say Sutton probably died elsewhere ... dumped along ... road...

It is obvious someone has been keeping him ... and probably ... exactly how he ... said a Homicide ... spokes...

Sutton was arrested ... ...

Informer 'probably killed'

A SYDNEY Coroner said yesterday it was likely a police informer and drug ad... ...utler was murdered.

...up $2 ...heroin from two ...shortly before he ...after a second inquest into the death of Dale Cather...Payne of Sydney.
...eged Ho... He said he won...people wanted to ...tioning in co... Attorney-G... the incident side...

He said p...

...e said for-... ...arcotics agents, ...Peter Marzol, ...ally the Det ...Sgt Ron ... the NSW office ...Payne's death, ...hey had been less ...han asked a ...first inquest if they ...anyone who might ...wished to harm...

The methadone solution

$4-MIL CITY OFFICE DRUG HAUL

By JOHN SILIC

POLICE claim to have smashed a major drug ring following the seizure of heroin worth $4 million in a raid on an office in Sydney's central business...

Hero!

... ...

Woman drug addict sent to prison

A woman who began to use heroin about 18 months ago and claimed to have been addicted for about a year was sentenced to jail when she appeared in the ACT Supreme Court yesterday.

Miss Karen Elizabeth McLeod, 22, unemployed, of Bailey Place, Yarralumla, pleaded guilty to aiding and ... breaking, entering and ...

In a statement to police, Miss McLeod had said that she had developed a habit costing about $300 a day. As she earned about $500 a fortnight in her job, she was heavily in debt to the person who was supplying the drugs, and as owed him about $5,000. In an attempt to get money, she had got the idea of robbing a takeaway shop.

On Wednesday, Crown prosecutor Mr Bernie Cleary told the court that ...

based on simple justice. Moreover, since it is finance that enables organised crime to continue operations despite arrests, the power to confiscate suspected profits and even assets connected with drug crime may significantly disrupt criminal activities. At present the Commonwealth Customs Act enables all monies prima facie obtained by reason of the offenders' illicit drug trafficking to be forfeited. This could be extended to State Acts.

All users are themselves criminal, and so the normal lines of information between victim and police are closed. Collection of information from informants, suspects and police Australia-wide is a paramount need. However, inter-agency co-ordination is characterised more by rivalry than co-operation. Clearly, better understanding and regular liaison, secondment and exchange are vital.

The priority that police should give to dealing with those high up in the distribution pyramid presents difficult problems. Those lower down are more visible, and the temptation to deal with them instead is great. Moreover, the isolation of important distributors from users means that evidence and intelligence are hard to come by. At present, Commonwealth police alone are entitled to intercept telecommunications; this is limited to gaining evidence directly related to a particular offence. Many recommendations have emphasised the need to allow phone tapping, controlled by judicial warrant, by all police to gain general intelligence.

Police have often argued for far greater powers in this area. These include interception without a warrant, searches without a warrant, warrants by telephone, abolition of the right to silence in questioning suspected drug traffickers, no bail, and compulsory urinalysis or blood analysis for any person suspected of drug use. Their usefulness in some situations is undoubted. But such suggestions, made from the understandable perspective of the frustrated crime fighter, do not consider the far-reaching consequences. Indeed it has been argued that increased police activity is counter-productive, leading to more competition, higher prices, more organised distribution and a greater emphasis on high profit drugs like heroin. Further, police already have a great deal of authority and power which can be, and is, abused. The measures advocated would give police more powers, and create greater inroads into civil liberties. The criminal suspect's right to remain silent in the face of police questions, for example, already of little use in the face of modern techniques of interrogation, is of great symbolic importance. Can this country afford making inroads into it?

Many people, especially those agitated by media reporting, argue that drug pushers have forfeited the right to be treated as ordinary members of the community, that drug crimes are a special case for extended police powers. It is not clear why this should be so.

Question: Is rape a special case? Murder? Burglary? If not, when would they be?

Possession: should it be a crime?

Despite the recent trend in viewing users of illicit drugs sympathetically, a crime of possession does undoubtedly have advantages.

(a) Some potential users will be deterred. If the psycho-social hypothesis of drug use put forward in Chapter 2 is accepted, however, the deterrence effect will not be great.
(b) The crime enables authorities to pick up persons at risk of dependence and refer them to treatment early in their drug career. The interval between beginning drug use and arrest, however, is usually two to five years, by which time drug habits are well entrenched.
(c) Drug users are isolated from potential users. This 'contagion theory', related to the public health model of drug use, is of limited value. The average convicted possessor is already well entrenched in the drug community. It is largely neophytes who introduce drugs to non-users.
(d) It enables police to keep in touch with the drug scene.
(e) It enables prosecution of traffickers where actual supply is difficult to prove.
(f) It is of great symbolic value, representing society's disapproval. This social sanction is of considerable importance in discouraging drug use early on, and would be significantly undercut if the disapproved product were legal.

There are, however, costs to the crime of possession. The offence has not worked in controlling drug abuse. The effect has been to label a large number of people 'criminal', thus limiting their educational and employment potential, and socially isolating them. (Conviction for marijuana possession prevents entry into law, medicine or the public service for life.) The root causes of drug use are thus merely exacerbated. It would be more effective if the reason for the continuation of classifying possession as crime were re-evaluated. If its symbolic value is of most importance, consideration should be given to alternative ways of expressing societal displeasure, as for example happens with tobacco and pornography.

Prison is largely seen as unsuitable for those whose only crime is possession. It steeps the user further in the criminal sub-culture, it is an ineffective deterrent to compulsive users, and it is an unsatisfactory environment in which to attempt rehabilitation. Rehabilitation services in prison are almost non-existent.

Attention has recently centred on the use of courts in assessing the drug use problem of those arrested, and if relevant diverting them from the criminal justice system to various treatment options. One option is diversion pre-trial. This is especially useful for young offenders, but the extent to which it is valid before guilt has been proven must be considered. The second option, favoured in Australia, operates merely between conviction and sentence. This may or may not be long enough to make an assessment of the person's drug use background. Certainly no proper treatment can be provided in such a short time.

Another possible diversion scheme may follow the third option, operating as a kind of sentence. We must be willing to invoke other alternatives, such as prison, if full assessment indicates that treatment is unsuitable or refused. The spectre of prison is a strong motivation for some to undergo treatment, and treatment without motivation will fail. However, as Victorian courts have held, no sentence should be imposed which, merely to induce acceptance of treatment, would be greater than that justified were treatment unavailable.

The effect of such diversion is treatment under coercion. Is this ethical? Voluntary behaviour is always relative; pressure from family or employer to undertake treatment is accepted by society, yet significant amounts of coercion are involved.

If society feels justified in invoking measures of social control, like prison, then it may well be justified in invoking treatment as an alternative. The justification is obviously greater in relation to, for example, drink drivers, or drug users who break and enter, than in relation to those whose only crime is drug use. Less justified still may be the belief that society is entitled to compulsorily treat people who are drug dependent but who have not been convicted of any crime. This is the situation in Singapore. Diversion has proved partially successful in lowering reconviction rates. However, society should be cautious in forcing different behaviour on unwilling victims. Social commentators in recent years have emphasised the need for doctors to resist paternalism, and respect the individual's right not to be 'cured'.

Question: Soviet psychiatric hospitals and 'the clockwork orange' are both forms of diversion and assessment. Are we going the same way? How will Australian schemes differ?

Cannabis
We have been regularly using cannabis as a case study of drug use in Australia, as an example of an unresolved issue. In this section, we deal specifically with the type of cannabis mixed in marijuana cigarettes. Other forms of the drug—Buddha sticks, hashish, hashish oil—contain more concentrated forms of the active component tetrahydrocannabinol (THC).

Many of the arguments raised for and against the crime of possession are relevant here. The main arguments in favour of legalisation are:

(a) The drug is probably no worse than alcohol or tobacco. The serious health dangers of these should, however, be remembered. Those who argue that 'if we can't handle those two, why should we legalise a third?' often ignore the ineffectiveness of the present law and the social costs it entails.
(b) The law is at present selectively enforced. Legal records show that cannabis smokers who are young, poor or unemployed are more often arrested, sometimes repeatedly. Older people and the middle class use the drug with virtual immunity. Significant disrespect for the law and suspicion of police are being engendered amongst a large section of society.
(c) The validity of the views that cannabis leads to crime, and that it is a stepping stone to hard drugs, has been strongly challenged.
(d) The present law may be increasing heroin use. There is some evidence that a shortage of cannabis encourages some of these

users to progress to heroin. At present, both drugs are linked together by their common criminality.
(e) The present law allows significant involvement by organised crime.

Against this, apart from arguments already raised in relation to possession, it is true that knowledge of the effect of long-term use is incomplete, conflicting and voluminous. This raises the basic policy question: to what extent should we control a product because of the possible long-term effects on heavy users? Cannabis is a significant danger to drivers and those in industry due to the loss of psychomotor control. Some argue that a solution may be a cannabis equivalent to the breathalyser. Such a device does not at present exist.

One of the main problems is that a change in the law may be seen as connoting government approval. Many people fear a large increase in use were cannabis laws to be changed.

There are various options for control.

(a) Status quo: Doing nothing has significant social costs. The Williams and Woodward commissions suggest that at least those convicted of a use-only crime should have their conviction destroyed after two years.
(b) Legalisation or decriminalisation of possession for personal use: These two options are not the same. The former allows possession, whilst the latter still penalises it, but merely by the imposition of fines which do not appear on a criminal record. Decriminalisation is thus less of a change, and does not indicate so great a reversal in public attitude, for it is argued that the symbolic tolerance of cannabis in either policy will greatly increase use and abuse. This has not been the US experience. However, if traffickers are still to be punished, there is a problem in proving non-personal use. Moreover, if use is not a criminal offence, how serious an offence can supply be? Who is a criminal? Thus either proposal may be largely an interim measure, getting rid of some evils of the present law and enabling reassessment before any further change is instituted.
(c) The same could be said for Sackville's suggestion to allow people to 'grow their own'. However, the amount harvested for two people's moderate use would be a traffickable

quantity, so enforcement against suppliers would be hard. Nevertheless, this remains a simple, attractive option. It does not signify public approval, while significantly undercutting the illicit market.

(d) State monopoly: This is likely to be unacceptable as it symbolises state approval. The effect will be, however, to undercut illicit markets and control distribution. It does not allow competing sellers to encourage increased drug use as has happened, for example, with tobacco.

(e) A licensing system: This proposal advocates a scheme similar to that currently operating with respect to some poisons, and to that which formerly operated in Sweden with respect to alcohol. Purchasers must sign for a limited quantity of the drug from licensed sellers. Moreover, a computer system could ensure that no one could purchase weekly more than a moderate supply. This scheme would not connote government approval and would enable control. It would also undercut the illcit market although not completely, as rationing systems always encourage black markets. Since cannabis is not physically addictive, it would strongly discourage heavy use.

Summary

In deciding among control measures, it must be remembered that most young people will not use cannabis or heroin, legal or not, and most users are experimental or casual, doing little harm to themselves or others. Heavy drug use is of concern in this area as elsewhere. Any change must be accompanied by public education about the dangers of drug use and also to counteract the misinformation that has developed. Research into alcohol has shown that gradual changes in the law do not greatly affect consumption. Above all, no law alone will stamp out drug abuse. Law makers must have realistic aims, and must decide the reasons for laws in concert with policy makers, politicians and the community.

Licit drugs

General

The greatest area of hope in curbing abuse of legal drugs lies in education. One of the main barriers to further control is the amount of taxes gained from alcohol and tobacco. Governments are therefore reluctant to discourage trade and so denude their own coffers. Indeed governments actively encourage trade in these drugs by large subsidies to the industries. Tobacco growing is being phased out, but tobacco trading is not. However, some legal measures are socially possible, and the success in reducing suicides by packaging sedatives differently indicates they can be successful.

(a) Reporting by pharmacists to a central supply agency, of the details of narcotics prescribed, may aid in the detection of over-prescribing doctors, and the discovery of addicts gaining prescriptions from a number of sources.

(b) Barbiturates may be banned or their use greatly restricted as they are of limited use medically and are over-represented among suicides and overdoses. Although they are not a common drug of abuse, there is a subgroup of habitual drug users whose drug of choice is barbiturates.

(c) Changes should be made in labelling laws to provide clear warnings on all drugs about their dangers especially in association with alcohol.

(d) Evidence is increasing that passive smoking is dangerous. Moves to prevent use in most areas of public buildings are under way.

(e) Random breath testing and drink–driver treatment diversion have been successful, but these and similar proposals raise civil liberty arguments.

(f) There is some potential in the fitting of mechanical devices to stop those with a blood alcohol content from starting their cars. However most of the current systems can be readily avoided and more research is needed.

(g) Arguments are often raised about the need for tighter controls over volatile substances. Given the huge range of household goods which can be sniffed or swigged, the solution is social and educational, not legal.

Advertising
The advertising of prescribed drugs to doctors could be more tightly controlled. The present system of gimmicks and sales pitches is an invitation to over-prescribing and a reinforcement of the need to treat by drugs. Whether alcohol and tobacco

advertising should be more restricted is a vexed question. Evidence on the effect of advertising bans is equivocal. The companies themselves argue that advertisements are merely to encourage brand loyalty by established users. If this were so, if all advertising were banned, why would users be less loyal? Alcohol and tobacco taking are habits begun in childhood. Advertising does influence children's behaviour. So no education program will succeed if there is continual negative reinforcement by advertising, movies, etc. A total advertising ban on the products may therefore be justified. Alcohol and tobacco are of economic benefit to Australia, but the costs they create virtually balance this. Certainly, as Baume said, the current self-regulatory code is 'inadequate'. Today's advertisements for alcohol and tobacco are clearly targeted at young women; health surveys, and presumably market research, show that this is the one expanding pool of users.

Sponsorship
Tobacco and alcohol advertising has recently moved strongly into the field of sports sponsorship. The danger with this is that sports figures are effective role models for young people. The concept of sports people simultaneously promoting health and cigarettes is ironic.

It has been suggested that the government should not give grants to organisations accepting alcohol or tobacco support and that levies be imposed on their advertising to pay for health promotion. Further, what would the effect of a ban on all such sponsorship be? The use of other companies in the area of sponsorship is untapped, but other companies may not completely fill the hiatus. Major issues are involved:

(a) Should governments continue to willingly step aside as supporters of sport and culture in favour of private companies? Moreover, it should be remembered that such sponsorship is tax deductible, and so the government is already paying for almost half the costs of sponsorship.
(b) What is the point of sport? If it is to encourage a healthy life for most of the population, do expensive presentations encourage participants, or spectators? If the point of sport is entertainment, to what extent should we accept that a cost of high quality entertainment is increased sickness and alcoholism?

Price and availability

Attention in recent years has been given to attempts to decrease overall alcohol consumption. Drew (1981) has argued that we need to question this approach, and concentrate instead on positive programs specifically related to alcohol abuse and drug use problems. The effectiveness of measures controlling price and availability is unclear. Perhaps in Australia different methods could be instituted in different States to study the problem properly. Sudden price rises seem to be more effective than gradual ones. However, evidence on whether this affects the long-term consumption pattern of heavy drinkers is not conclusive. Maintenance of a real price for alcohol in proportion to income has seemed to have an effect on consumption levels. This would in consequence make low alcohol beer cheaper, but the barriers to LA beer are largely social and psychological; recent advertising may have helped alter this, in respect of merely social drinkers at least. There is no clear relationship between drinking levels and either the number of outlets or times of opening. If alcohol was less available in social settings, however, there may be an impact on heavy drinkers, because of the contextual and structural restraints on drinking.

What can be concluded is that further research is needed; cost increases if implemented should be significant, and explained to consumers to gain their support; target groups need to be identified. Different measures will affect different groups. Problem drinking of all sorts is essentially a social problem. Community attitudes are the vital ingredient in the causes and solutions of licit drug problems. As ever, the use of legal controls over drugs can only be secondary to social change.

Question: A Geraldton publican was charging Aborigines $5 a middy. Do you approve? Will it work?

The present and the future

The distinctions between control and treatment are often blurred. Both see the drug taking as the crucial problem, and the drug-related behaviour as secondary. Options for compulsory treatment beg the questions of what is crime and what is sickness. Tables 19 and 20 list the drugs against which police action can be taken. By definition, according to our social taboos, treatment cannot be offered for the results of abuse of these drugs (see Table 3, on cannabis use); although, more recently, detoxification and treatment units are now more viable since they do not have to report their clients to the police.

Table 19
Criminal charges associated with specific drugs 1977-81

Drug type	1977	1978	1979	1980	1981
Cannabis	17 978	14 249	17 501	20 278	26 506
Narcotics	3 676	4 262	3 520	2 611	3 745
Amphetamines	155	123	245	201	624
Barbiturates/hypnotics	784	503	907	630	342
Hallucinogens	232	286	278	290	263
Tranquillisers	86	193	248	220	263
Antidepressants	3	5	13	5	2
Other drugs	110	327	159	280	202
Total	23 024	19 948	22 871	24 515	31 947

Source: Australian Federal Police, published in Australia, Department of Health, *Statistics on drug abuse in Australia*

In Table 19 we see the great diversion of legal resources to handling cannabis use; while any interpretation of the misuse of prescription drugs, which make up most of the rest of the charges, is fraught with social problems. Are these polydrug users? Addicts resulting from hospital procedures? Or pharmacy burglaries? Table 20 shows remarkable changes in drugs seized in Australia over the years. Do today's figures reflect changing social usage, indeed an epidemic, or improved police efficiency, or increased social condemnation of drug use? Or all three?

That the future will see even more changes is clear. Law Reform Commissions in many States are working on new answers. It may be of value here to turn to the recommendations of a national Drug Summit and a national drug workshop (Appendixes 2 and 1 to Chapter 11) to see the position of the country on control measures when the meetings were held. The recommendations reflect a trend

Table 20
Seizures of selected drugs by Federal agencies 1977-83

Type of drug		1977	1978	1979	1980	1981	1982	1983
Heroin	(kg)	11.7	17.9	29.3	7.9	9.5	32.0	97.1
Cocaine	(g)	140	—	178	6964	311	8925	8797
Cannabis oil	(kg)	37.2	97.7	54.2	108.3	2.8	30.4	60.1
Cannabis[a]	(kg)	704.0	7648.0	554.1	581.0	1728.9	2499.7	1665.4

a: Includes tops, seeds and resin and other
Source: Australian Federal Police, published in Australia, Department of Health, *Statistics on drug abuse in Australia*

towards greater control of the use of licit drugs (lower and lower permissible alcohol levels while driving, for instance), and recognition that the law has a comparatively minor part to play in the long-term control of illicit drugs, which must be, in the end, a matter of social control.

Nevertheless for many people, because of their values, social perspective or personal experiences, legal control will remain the favoured policy option. Where this is so it will affect all four of the usual avenues of response, as indicated in Table 21, so that teacher and doctor see their roles as controlling student and patient for their own good, just as fines and imprisonment are imposed for the social good. Punishment is seen as an effective deterrent, and as retribution on behalf of the rest of the citizenry.

Table 21
Framework for drug issues 5: control as policy

	Avenues of approach			
	Control	Treatment	Education	Social change
Policy	Exert controls on supply of and demand for drugs			
Aspects of strategy:				
Physical states	Restraints for suppliers and users	Sedation, replacement therapy	Instruct on harm done by drugs	Reduce all drug outlets
Ethical goals	Suppliers and users forfeit citizen rights	Medical control of treatment	Teacher control of classroom	Reimpose strict standards of behaviour
Aesthetic responses	Drug use hidden, amoral	Treatment should be nasty	School should be tough	Drugs are nasty
Social rules	Accept police right of intrusion and surveillance	Treatment should be punitive	School rules should be firm, users expelled	Increase reliance on laws
Individual perspective	I'll try hard to hide my drug use			

7
Treatment

Public and private

Treatment is only one avenue of response to drug abuse, although to many it is the only option; for many people, those who abuse drugs are obviously 'sick'. To some extent treatment overlaps with control, as we have discussed previously, in that all treatment and rehabilitation services are concerned not only with care for the individual users but ultimately with returning individuals to a 'normal' life and therefore with maintaining social order and stability.

Treatment in relation to drug abuse implies more than a purely medical response, with cure as the goal. As well as medical care it embraces social and individual support services, as in, for example, counselling, shelter and assistance with employment, and access to agencies which deal with the physiological, psychological and environmental aspects of drug problems. Treatment in this broad sense also includes rehabilitation (successful treatment solutions require long-term perspectives for enduring change) and prevention (early detection of drug use, or treatment of some of the precursors of abuse). It is counter-productive to regard all these as separate treatment services; rather they are part of the continuum of care that responds to problems of drug use and abuse.

There have been two classic models of drug treatment—from the perspectives of public health and private medicine respectively. Public health is the perspective which gives us ideas of hygiene and immunisation, and seeks identification of the host of the invading infection, the agent carrying the infection and the context or environment where it all happens. This is a common model within treatment agencies, where the drug is seen as the damaging agent, the client as the host and the environment as encouraging the invasion by the drug. This appraisal leads quickly to efforts to control: ban the drug and treat the drug abuser. The strengths of the public health approach are that practitioners can deal with the whole environment, reducing its support for drug abuse by legislation and law enforcement, as well as by altering social customs. Blood alcohol testing is a good example. Public health officers can also take an overview using statistical evidence and, linking evidence of use to biological principles, can contribute to policy. Disadvantages are the labelling of the drug user as 'the problem'; the risk that drug use is seen as infectious, as if it were typhoid or cholera; and the potential loss of the individual's viewpoint.

Private medicine assumes that diagnosis of the problem, and decision making on the treatment of choice, rest with the medical adviser, who thus determines the sufferer's needs and treats them according to medical standards of the day. The strengths of this are the ability to respond to each person's need for a drug and the individual response to that drug, and the confidentiality and high level of skill in the resultant care. Weaknesses are the potential labelling of the user as 'sick', and so not responsible for his/her actions. While the adviser retains responsibility for the cure, the drug abuser has a vested interest in not being cured but in persisting with chosen behaviour. Treatment offered as an alternative to gaol for heroin use falls into this category, and has not been noticeably successful. Other issues, which those offering treatment need to consider, are the tendency to apply one's own moral sanctions to drug use and so to 'blame the victim' and the risk of labelling the patient by the disease of drug abuse and so missing the multifaceted nature of drug use.

Looking at treatment from the point of view of our totems and taboos theme, it is clear that the approaches chosen reflect society's conflicting attitudes to the subject of drug abuse. There is a taboo about facing the real causes of abuse, a taboo which forbids recognition of our less than ideal world, our family conflicts, and our double standards, all of which may well be behind the original drug use. Instead the emphasis is on the drug abuser as being a defaulter from the totems of our society, the breaker of rules, the wrongdoer, the deviant. The taboo forbids any thought that the problems may be due to the structure or nature of society. Hence, treatment may be offered by society as a humane gesture to pull the 'victims' out of their misery, but it is equally likely to be offered out of concern for the maintenance of social order and stability, for the maintenance of the totems.

Such a response is reflected in the way that treatment has been made available. It is generally agreed that services have been poorly funded and under-resourced. Partly because of this they have been fragmented, competitive, unco-ordinated, selective in whom they treat and limited in what they offer. There has been no adequate data collection of existing resources, the type of clients who present, the problems presented or the outcomes. Evaluation of methods has been practically non-existent and has rarely been allowed for in funding grants. These characteristics of drug treatment agencies are markedly different from those for more socially acceptable diseases, for instance hospitals and health centres, where equipment is usually of the finest and research grants are available. The result, not surprisingly, is a difficulty in obtaining staff, and low morale in many agencies.

Objectives of treatment

Underlying the choice of approach to treatment is the decision on whether the treatment should aim for a drug-free existence, or whether it is sufficient to enable a drug abuser to become stabilised at a given level of use. Answers to this question ultimately determine the treatment services provided and the community expectations of their outcomes. They will depend on whether we seek to control society or trust the individual or try to do both.

There are widely differing views on this issue although there is growing acceptance that there are circumstances in which it is appropriate to prescribe controlled drugs to abusers, and where it is not realistic to expect a drug-free existence in the short term. Such circumstances are usually cases of long-term addiction to opioid substances (heroin) where repeated attempts to give up drugs have failed. While maintenance programs are offered in Australia, there are also services that aim for a drug-free state at the end of treatment.

It is becoming clear that no single treatment will provide the whole solution. Drug abuse is complex, with users on a continuum from the occasional experimenter to the compulsive addict with a prolonged history of addiction. Many substances are involved and they in turn vary in the degree of harm they cause. Also an increasing number of drug users are multiple drug users. Not all individuals with drug problems suffer from drug dependence. For a minority drug taking is sometimes a facet of a serious personality disorder or even of a mental illness. There is considerable disagreement about the existence of a uniform personality or type of person who becomes either an addict or an individual with drug problems. Too often there has been a collapsing together of drug use patterns in the urgent rush to find a broad explanation/solution.

Each individual drug misuser's problems need to be assessed and the best match made to appropriate services. There needs to be a clear distinction drawn in this assessment between those problems which preceded the person's drug use (problems of origin) and those problems which are the outcome of drug use (problems of consequence). Strategies targeted at a problem of origin, such as poor family relations, will be inappropriate for dealing with problems of consequence, such as chronic criminality. Unless both sets of problems are dealt with we cannot expect significant changes in the drug user's behaviour. For some a medical response will be appropriate, for others a social work response might be more suited. For yet others, counselling by a teacher or health educator might be the best response. No single discipline can cope alone and there is a need for collaboration between various services and disciplines. Such collaboration requires a network of co-ordinated agencies operating with a long-term perspective.

It is important that clients are assessed before treatment commences (that is, we should identify the extent, pattern and characteristics of drug abuse). Most treatment modes have high drop-out rates in early stages and many addicts try a variety of services before they find a suitable mode or become totally disillusioned with treatment and give up. Complete and thorough assessment is time consuming and does sometimes present practical problems for practitioners. Nevertheless better assessment would avoid the trial and error approach and result in a better use of limited resources. Perhaps there is a need for independent referral groups who can fulfil the assessment function and refer to appropriate agencies.

Types of treatment

There are no miracle modes of treatment and rehabilitation although new developments are often touted as 'the' solution. Proponents of particular treatment modes are often convinced that their approach is the only one. A range of services have evolved to treat drug misuse and dependence in Australia. These are briefly outlined below.

Detoxification/withdrawal
This service may be given in hospital or as an outpatient. The aim is to eliminate physical dependence on drugs such as heroin or alcohol under expert supervision. This is considered a humane means of allowing patients who have a severe addiction to

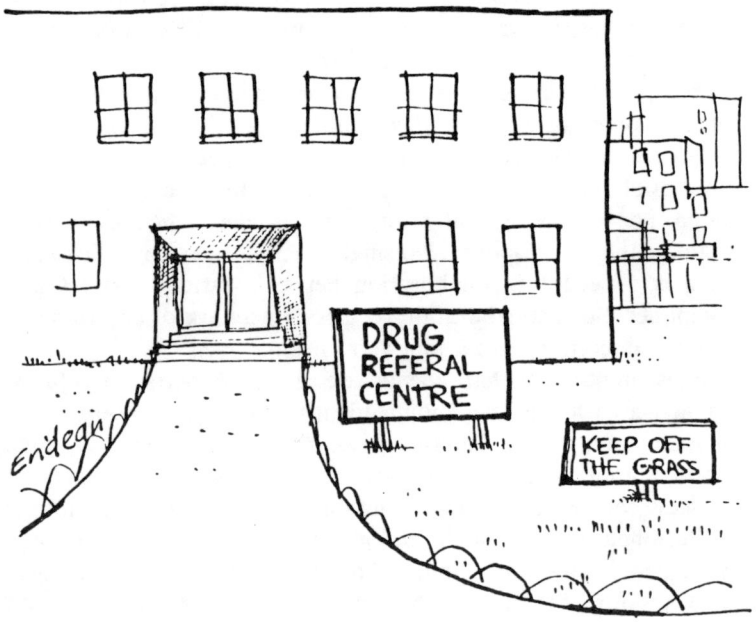

Cartoon by Endean, reprinted by permission of the artist, from **Bulletin**, *29 May 1979*

withdraw from their drug, at least temporarily, and of bringing some order into their lives as well as attracting them to long-term treatment. There is general consensus, however, that detoxification from any drug abuse is of limited value without longer-term support, and help to change environment and/or lifestyle.

Therapeutic communities
These are full-time residential drug-free communities. They are highly organised and provide peer group support, group therapy, counselling and job functions. They provide a protected structured environment within which social and sobriety skills can be learnt. Quite apart from anything else, they offer time 'off the street'. Their basic goal is to persuade the drug abusers to abandon antisocial and self-destructive behaviours and pursue a mature and productive way of life. They have a high drop-out rate in the early stage of treatment. In Australia there are therapeutic communities in most States, largely run by non-government agencies. They are often criticised for their self-selection and high drop-out rates in early stages of treatment, but for some people this mode is the most suited.

Narcotics Anonymous/Alcoholics Anonymous (NA/AA)
These are fellowships of recovering addicts who rely on self-help and support by others who have similar experiences. At the beginning of the NA/AA process, it is asked that the member accept that the addiction is out of control and that life has become unmanageable. Thereafter there is a twelve-step program. Many addicts find the atmosphere of acceptance and understanding, with people with whom they can identify, much easier to accept than treatment from expert counsellors who have not themselves been addicted. There is evidence from USA to suggest that peer support programs are very powerful aids in a whole range of social problems including drugs, alcohol, compulsive gambling and child abuse.

Outpatient drug-free programs
These provide treatment for abusers of opiates and other drugs in various programs that differ widely in duration, goals and content. They include individual, group, family or other therapy, highly organised daytime therapeutic communities, drug care programs,

recreational activities and counselling. Their major advantage is that they are cheap and allow the client to live a normal life. Their disadvantage is that they do not prevent client access to drugs.

Drug replacement programs
The currently controversial example of replacing one drug by another is the substitution of methadone for heroin. Methadone maintenance is only one part of the array of potential treatment responses, many of which are potentially complementary, e.g. NA/AA or a therapeutic community to follow detoxification. Many methadone maintenance programs in their present form would have much to gain from incorporating the concepts of peer support and self-help. It is apparent however that drug users cannot be expected to go from the street into a social vacuum.

Methadone maintenance was introduced in Australia in the 1970s. Methadone is usually provided in outpatient settings (specialist clinics) with high level daily doses. Doses vary from blockade levels with a high enough dosage to eliminate any 'buzz' from taking heroin, to lower dosage which still permits a buzz from heroin. Time in treatment varies, with most clients staying for more than a year, and the risk is that it may be for a lifetime. When combined with rehabilitation and counselling methadone maintenance enables clients to change their lifestyles.

Methadone maintenance as a treatment is still subject to debate. The major areas of dispute are the idea of using an addictive substance to treat heroin, substituting one addiction for another, concern about the danger of methadone leaking into illegal channels, and the long-term effects on health. A major disadvantage with methadone maintenance is that like most outpatient services it only partly takes the client out of the drug scene. It does not replace the peer group, nor does it assist with strong support even when there is counselling available. The rationale for methadone maintenance is that addiction is a chronic and relapsing condition so it is unrealistic to aim for a drug-free solution for everyone within a specific period. By substituting methadone there is time for a heroin addict to resume a normal life, which leads to other advantages such as reduced mortality and criminal behaviour and increased well-being, and continued contact with the treatment agency. The National Health and Medical Research Council has accepted the use of methadone maintenance in certain cases where abstinence is impossible in the short term.

Other services
In addition to the treatment modes detailed above there are a variety of other interventions that need to be provided to meet drug abusers' problems. These include:
(a) long-term residential facilities for people undergoing rehabilitation and who require intensive physical and psychological care
(b) short-term residential care to avoid imminent relapse to drug-using lifestyle and to follow up detoxification
(c) halfway houses, emergency accommodation
(d) outreach programs to reach those unaware of, or unwilling to seek, help
(e) drop-in centres and shopfronts where drug users can obtain counselling, information and legal advice and where contact can be made in the early stages of drug use.

Does treatment work?

The answer to this question depends on what has been accepted as the aim of treatment. Early evaluations (pre 1970s) of treatment modes were pessimistic about the high rates of relapse as expectations had been for total abstinence. Those who hold this view will always regard anything less than total abstinence as failure. The two case studies, extracted from clinical records, demonstrate that 'cure' is not an appropriate word for the interaction between clinician and patient in the drug field.

Current treatment programs and measures of success concentrate not only on drug use but also on remedying the associated adverse social, behavioural and health effects. In addition expectations have been modified in the light of increasing awareness of the chronic and relapsing nature of the problem.

The present view of treatment is that it is associated with favourable outcomes. Recent studies point to the success of three commonly used modes (methadone maintenance, therapeutic communities and outpatient drug-free programs) in reducing drug use and antisocial behaviour and in improving job prospects.

> **Case Study 1**
>
> I am recovering from heroin addiction. I am a woman, 38 years old, a university graduate in biochemistry. I worked fourteen years as a clinical biochemist. Ten of those years in clinical toxicology —the detection and measurement of licit and illicit drugs in human biological specimens—in a large teaching hospital.
>
> I have drunk alcohol and smoked marijuana since I was 21 and I was 'normal' as far as drug use went. If anything, I felt superior to the 'weak drug addicts'—society's refuse—whose names and specimens I dealt with on a daily basis.
>
> At 28, I began to experiment with heroin, methadone and various other narcotics. I was an addict on the street for eighteen months. I went to Odyssey House after an accidental overdose of barbiturates (taken during an attempt to withdraw from heroin), and left after two years.
>
> I went on drinking alcohol and smoking marijuana on a 'social' basis, but five years later I again picked up heroin. This time I went to Rozelle Hospital. Since January 1984 [written in January 1985] I have been drug and alcohol free and going to Narcotics Anonymous.

For those who see treatment success in terms of a drug-free state the situation is less favourable. Fewer than 10 per cent of people entering treatment services remain drug free over the ensuing years which is about the same rate suggested for those who spontaneously revert to a drug-free life.

A critical element in treatment success is individual motivation; for individuals to benefit they must accept responsibility for changing their lives rather than being passive patients receiving a cure. Most do not come without some form of coercion—usually the law, peers or the family. Other factors that promote successful treatment seem to be the establishment of rapport between counsellor and client to provide support and influence, and the length of time spent by the client in treatment (generally the longer the time the better the outcome).

Evaluation of treatment services
Evaluation of treatment services is essential for the community to know whether treatment services are effective, and which treatment modes are successful for which problems. Agencies need to set realistic goals in light of the recalcitrant nature of the problem, particularly when dealing with heroin addiction. It may not be realistic to set a drug-free state as a short-term goal. Success might

---

Case Study 2

I am a 37-year-old teacher in Tertiary Education. I was a drug addict for twelve years and it is eleven months since I last used a drug.

My understanding of an addict is not someone who uses addictive drugs, but someone who cannot stop using mood-altering substances by means of personal will.

Almost two years ago, as I lay in bed in detox at the beginning of my recovery, the bed on one side was occupied by an alcoholic, on the other side was a Serepax addict, and across the aisle was a barbiturate addict. For those of us who recover it is all the same disease regardless of the legality of the mode of supply.

When I started using cannabis, I could not understand why it was illegal and alcohol was legal, fifteen years later I still cannot. Later, when I began to experiment with heroin, I was encouraged by the thought 'if they were wrong about cannabis, they are probably wrong about this too'.

Early in my using, I noticed that my dependence on drugs was quite total, while other social users around me could take it or leave it. I am an addict, they are not, no amount of prohibition by me personally or by the state through legislation could alter my pattern of using until I was sufficiently desperate.

When I was using I waited with desperation for the day when heroin would be supplied to registered addicts, yet I believe that if this had happened I would still be using. I sometimes bought methadone on the black market when I could not obtain heroin. I can remember this program being regarded as a total farce by most people who had anything to do with it.

be better defined in measures aimed at reducing the adverse effects of drug abuse, for example achievement or partial achievement of such favourable outcomes as a drug-free lifestyle, a narcotic-free lifestyle, reduced antisocial behaviour (such as crime), improved employment status, reduced mortality, better physical and emotional health and improved self-image. Consistent evaluation will eventually lead to better results in terms of matching concerns to interventions. The whole range of evidence—physical, social, ethical, and aesthetic—needs to be considered in the evaluation. The long-term outcome of the strategy applied cannot be predicted without knowledge of social norms and goals in which the treatment is taking place. Part of the evaluation should also be from the perspective of the client, as the two case studies show.

Voluntary non-government agencies
These agencies play a significant role in providing treatment services. They have a degree of flexibility and responsiveness to client needs that official agencies cannot emulate. In addition they draw on reserves of expertise and dedication while providing a link to the wider grass roots community. They do not suffer the taint of authority that dissuades some drug addicts from attending official institutions. Richmond Fellowship, Salvation Army (Mancare Community) and other religious agencies, while not basically giving treatment, provide valuable services.

Future directions

At any one time several agencies may be involved in working with a drug user; health departments, child welfare, probation and parole are the most common but specific medical practitioners, police, voluntary welfare organisations and other groups may also be involved. Routinely some drug users will play off one drug agency against another. Even when this does not occur agencies with different mandates tend to function at cross purposes. A very disturbing example of this is the recycling of drug users from prison back into the community without adequate liaison or preparation. The consequences for the community are that unco-ordinated services lead to action that is largely ineffective. Case co-ordination requires a great deal of close co-operation between agencies; policy needs to develop to encourage this to occur.

The needs of treatment staff must be properly met if treatment programs are to improve. Some frequently mentioned difficulties are staff 'burn out', lack of training and poor job prospects in a disorganised service. Remedies that might improve the situation are:

(a) the provision of specific training in recognition of the specialist nature of the work
(b) reorganisation of services to develop a career structure, possibly via integration of drug treatment services into the general health care system
(c) rotation of staff to avoid stress, to help preserve work satisfaction and to build up a pool of experience
(d) use of specialist consultants particularly in those services provided by non-government organisations.

Recommendations from DA:NA (see Chapter 11, Appendix 1), and their results in terms of the $65 million disbursed by the subsequent political Summit, are, as with law enforcement, an indication for future directions. In the event, the money from the National Campaign Against Drug Abuse was allotted as follows: National Media Campaign—$5 million; treatment—$15 million nationally for each of the next three years; and education $5 million for each of the next three years.

It is worth noting that the recommendations on resources and treatment were made in relation to a general statement that alcohol and nicotine were the major drugs of abuse in Australia, and should have first call on priorities for research and treatment. They reflect the rather paltry conditions under which treatment agencies must work in Australia, the controversial nature of methadone treatment, and the marked difference between the drugs area and the power of mainstream medical treatments such as surgery. The field clearly needs policy directions and strategies of its own. Action plans which have been successful are discussed and listed in Part 3 on Action. Here we might summarise criteria essential to a successful treatment strategy.

(a) The treatment must be congruent with the drug user's cultural experience. Alcoholics Anonymous has been accepted worldwide because the principle of self-help is congruent with people's beliefs. The user must be able to return to his environment drug free.

(b) The treatment must be congruent with the cultural expectations of the wider society. There is much disagreement about the use of methadone as a treatment, however its use is approved by many because it frees the addicted person from criminality and is therefore good for the restoration of social order.

(c) The treatment programs should be targeted at empowering the drug user as a person who wishes to change. A satisfactory way of feeling about oneself is a real need. A treatment which brings about a state of helplessness will not be satisfactory.

Question: Looking from your particular perspective on treatment, what do you think would be an 'appropriate' procedure for treating heroin dependence during pregnancy?

Examples of existing treatment agencies are listed in Chapter 12, 'A national repertoire of action plans'.

In conclusion, we can review the position with regard to treatment much as we did at the close of the previous chapter on control. The appendices to Chapter 11 supply the lists of recommendations for the future directions of treatment of drug abuse in Australia, and Table 22 summarises the implications of choosing treatment to be the dominant strategy for reducing abuse. Just as a control strategy implied that compulsory treatment is justified, a treatment strategy suggests that rehabilitation is an essential element of a prison sentence, and that drug users should be separated within schools, and sent to counsellors and medical officers. A drug user, being potentially sick, should not be blamed but treated.

The public health approach would approve of segregation of drug abusers (to prevent contagion) and cautionary instruction of the population (so that they avoid the risks).

Table 22
Framework for drug issues 6: treatment as policy

	Avenues of approach			
	Control	Treatment	Education	Social change
Policy	Treatment of supplier and user as sick			
Aspects of strategy: Physical states	Needs supervision	Diagnosis of physical damage	Teach physical damage from drug use	Large hospital drug wards
Ethical goals	Supervision only for treatment purposes	Cure available to all	Protect students from contagion	Drug users are not to be blamed
Aesthetic responses	Clean up the mess	Treatment is white and clean	Keep schools white and clean	Tidy drug users away
Social rules	Prison must rehabilitate	Drug user is sick	Refer drug users to doctor, counsellor	Drug use must be contained
Individual perspective	If I like my drug I won't want to be cured			

8
Education

Voyages of discovery

Education would be the preferred option for most people when it comes to preventing drug abuse. Personal responsibility for drug taking and wise use of necessary drugs are, in our conventional wisdom, the best options we can hope for. It is education, within the family, within schools, in higher education and in the community to which we look for correct information and help in learning to use that information wisely. Unfortunately, education is also often the too hard basket, the catch-all, and the place of last resort. Information exchanged without the skills to change attitudes is not educational, and those skills may or may not be part of a teacher's standard repertoire.

Standardised views of education vary from the outmoded 'jug and bottle' view of knowledge, where information is transmitted by the teachers as if into an inert row of vessels waiting to receive it; through the master-apprentice view, where the teacher has a great deal of wisdom which he or she shares daily with the student; to the 'we are explorers together' view of recently established progressive schools. Clearly, drug education would differ markedly, when delivered with each of these perspectives. In the first, one could hazard a guess that the harmful effects of some forbidden drugs would be all that would be mentioned—with the most forbidden not mentioned at all. An example of this approach might be the police lectures to schools, which gave many school children their first sight of a marijuana plant, or a heroin syringe. Alcohol and LSD were never mentioned. This is education seen as control, with mixed messages which keep reality in the established totem-taboo framework.

In the master-apprentice perspective, we might instance the physical education classes, where physically fit models of non-drinking, non-smoking men and women urge their students to be as fit as they are and show them how the totem is the Olympic medal, and the taboo is the fat slob. This is close to treatment strategy in education: cure your unfitness by exercise and competitive sport. The third view is, in part or in whole, the preferred approach for most teachers in the health education curriculum, the area most likely to be charged with drug education in formal institutions. The 'we are discovering together' mode goes well with the general theme of self-development and personal responsibility, which is the case policy of most health education programs.

There is no doubt that prevention (intervention before drug abuse problems arise) in terms of Australian social values must be morally regarded as better than cure. On the other hand, many prevention measures, such as breath-alcohol testing and banning of nicotine advertising, conflict with other strong social values, such as freedom of individuals to take risks in their own way. Changes in social attitudes have been necessary to enable most of the stronger education measures to succeed; these are discussed further in the second section on prevention, social change (Chapter 9).

Education through formal institutions seems a non-threatening option for drug intervention in a society which values education, provides at least twelve years of it to all citizens and uses the educational system to enshrine social values. Education for self-development is a comparatively recent introduction into Australian schools, within the last two decades. Even more recent has been the movement into health and human relationships education. Adequate professional preparation is seldom provided for the teaching of these courses; most teacher preparation programs focus on specialist content areas, and on teaching skills rather than personal development. For those that do deal with personal development and change, there is a difficulty in drug education in that the very topic challenges social values.

Controversy has ebbed and flowed over the position of health education in relation to parental responsibilities and the school curriculum. Should it be directed or left to the values of parents

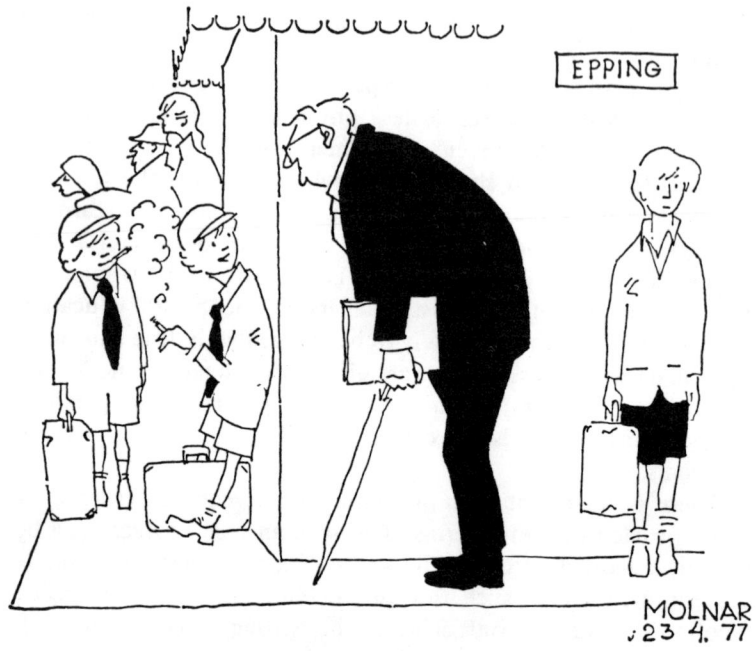

"It's all right, Dad. It's only pot."

Cartoon by Molnar, reprinted by permission of the artist, from *Sydney Morning Herald*, 23 April 1977

and teachers? Should it be a subject in its own right, or spread through the curriculum in history and literature as well as in physical education? In 1978 the national Curriculum Development Centre came down on both sides of the fence, outlining a firm Health Education curriculum (which included drug use), and recommending that the themes and issues should be discussed in other subject areas as well.

Schools around Australia instituted Health Education, Education for Living, Living Skills, Social Issues and Human Relationships programs, in any of which drug issues might be discussed, but which had widely differing guidelines and objectives. At the tertiary level, first diploma courses in Health Education and then degree courses in Canberra, Tasmania, Adelaide and Perth produced health educators with skills in drug education. But the total graduates a year would not exceed two hundred, in a national population of several million school children. Meanwhile, medical schools and other courses for health professionals rarely touched on drug education as a preventive measure. Rather the considerable time spent on learning about drugs would present them as a preferred option to surgery or to letting nature take its course. Two medical schools, Newcastle and Flinders, and several Colleges of Advanced Education such as Lincoln Institute in Melbourne, have developed courses with a community orientation on sound drug use, and prevention of abuse.

Two institutions in particular have provided centres for professional retraining and each of these has become involved in helping educators at schools and at professional levels to deal with drug-related and other issues. The University of New South Wales is host to the postgraduate Health Training Centre and the University of Melbourne to the now independent Social Biology Resources Centre.

The longest running drug education program in Australia is the National Drug Education Program, first endorsed by the Commonwealth, States and Territories of Australia in 1970 and given a new lease of life after the report of the Australian Royal Commission of Inquiry into Drugs in 1980. Immediate contacts are the Drugs of Dependence Branch of the Commonwealth Department of Health and the Alcohol and Drug Services of each State and Territory, who in general make up the management committee.

Educational strategy: the National Drug Education Program

Long-established and well-planned, the National Drug Education Program has developed clear statements of the nature and purposes of drug education, which we cannot do better than to quote. The Program, while on the one hand demonstrating what can be done in developing clear strategy, shows also the problem of a lack of related national policies on drug use and abuse, and the lack of comprehensive funding of the action levels of school, community and professional training. In the same fifteen years that the National Drug Education Program was developed there were, as we have noted previously, many commissions of inquiry into drugs. Few of the recommendations, even though almost unanimous, were implemented. So the National Drug Education Program remained a strategy without a policy to back it; and the hoped for connections with other interventions, such as educational skills for law enforcement agents and medical practitioners, have never eventuated.

Neither have policy decisions which would have led to changes in teacher training or even in teacher upgrading. Thus effective action plans were developed within the Program (see Chapter 12) but implemented only rarely.

Principles of drug education : key points

Drug education programs should be based on a knowledge of the factors which predispose, enable, and reinforce drug use in the community.

Education should proceed from what people already know, and should recognise that the level of existing knowledge will vary with the age and general educational level of the target group.

Drug education should be conducted for target groups in settings which are familiar to them, and should involve persons with whom the target group would normally have contact.

It should be recognised that risk taking can be an attractive aspect in regard to experimentation with and use of drugs, and that drug education programs therefore need to present alternatives to drug use.

Programs should be presented which have sequence, progression and continuity over a period of time.

Programs should address priorities, and should follow the sequence of analysis of needs, identification of target groups, setting of objectives, selection of the appropriate strategies and program evaluation.

Programs must necessarily involve recipients in their planning and implementation.

Educational approaches that rely on fear arousal are rarely appropriate. Similarly 'information only' approaches are generally not recommended.

Drug education should encompass practical information on drugs and their actions, the laws relating to drug use, and sources of information and assistance.

Educational messages in different programs should have a consistency and coherence with one another.

Programs should include strategies to reinforce and enable the desirable new drug use behaviour patterns.

Education resources (e.g. publications, audio-visuals, etc.) need to be thoroughly tested prior to general use.

These principles were intended to apply not only to high school programs, usually the target for concern about drugs and the focus for the cliché 'too little, too late'. They apply equally to primary schools, the elderly at risk of over-medication, doctors, pharmacists, nurses, journalists and industry.

Strategies in practice

These well-articulated objectives and associated funding have produced a wide range of curriculum packages with most imaginative programs and well-executed handbooks and classroom materials. 'Why Smoke?' and 'Broaden Your Options' are titles of such programs which indicate the type of values clarification, realistic approach which has had considerable success with high school students. Selling Us Ourselves was a package which allowed a teacher to analyse drug advertisements with the students, and students to identify the powerful social messages for themselves. The emphasis is again on values clarification and attitude change, the self-help approach which is a broad strategy direction becoming more and more common in Australian schools. Giving only detailed information on the drug itself has been shown by evaluation to be sadly effective in merely teaching the student how to take the drug.

A highly effective and well-targeted community education program was Pregnant Pause, designed to help the intending parent to face what is a very new social dilemma. As rates of nicotine and alcohol use by females climb steeply to match the male rates (and even exceed them in early high school years), this age-old taboo for women has clearly been lifted. This leaves women with a difficult personal decision to make about what has been previously enforced by social rules: the avoidance of drugs while pregnant, all of which cross the human placenta far more readily than in any other mammal. We learnt hideously from thalidomide; we are only just discovering the foetal alcohol syndrome, where the child of even a moderately alcoholic mother may be born with stereotyped abnormal features and severe mental retardation. Nicotine slows foetal heart rates and movement; there is some evidence that children of smoking mothers perform less well intellectually than those of non-smokers, and even harder evidence that the non-smoking children of smoking mothers have a higher mortality from cancer. Thus the challenge for educators to reach and to help the population of young female smokers is great. Such challenges are repeated for every special group listed in the objectives of the National Drug Education Program; so that while some broad strategy directions can be discerned in drug education, such as peer support, values clarification and improving decision-making skills, for many target groups the strategy needs to be custom-built from the broader repertoire of counselling techniques, behaviour modification, community development and social change techniques.

Another source of valuable education strategies is the self-development alternative which now abounds in our newsagencies and bookshops. One feels that market forces are well ahead of classic educational models here. Reputable and effective books, such as Berne's *Games people play*, and assertiveness training of all sorts provide self-education, self-help techniques which stand the individual in good stead in a world where totems and taboos are particularly likely to be in conflict with one another. For this reason it is worthwhile summarising some useful educational techniques. All are integral to drug education in that they allow teacher and students to challenge totems and taboos together, and allow each their own position of value and dignity.

Values clarification
A now slightly démodé technique whereby a situation of potential conflict is talked through by the participants, theoretically in an atmosphere of acceptance and trust. Examples are choosing items to take into a bomb shelter, choosing a team for that final desert island, 'what would you do if . . . your baby brother was shooting

smack?' The strengths are the chance to talk about taboo topics and find you are not alone. The weaknesses are the difficulty of ensuring trustworthy settings and the absence of guidelines or goals; some of the early authors in this field were Simon, Howe and Kirschenbaum.

Transactional analysis (TA)
An entertaining but most insightful method of applying Freudian psychoanalytic technique to oneself, for oneself. The strength is the ability it gives to replay old parental tapes, and review one's most ritualised behaviours. As a means of identifying totems and taboos accepted from parents, teachers and other authority figures it is excellent. First-class authors have translated TA for tots, teens and parents (Freed) and for just about everybody (James and Jongeward). The drawback is that TA is so generally used that it can become a recipe, or trivialised, or its power may be unrealised by an insensitive group leader. In general though, the ideas are sturdy enough to withstand misuse.

Effectiveness training
Techniques of problem solving were developed by Thomas Gordon, for use in parent, teacher and leadership effectiveness training. These allow the resolution of tough issues without loss of dignity. Concentrating on the common problem, they allow both sides to find common ground without the need to take up adversary positions. There are very comprehensive training programs which sometimes make this approach appear a narrow professional tool, but Gordon's manuals are good value by themselves.

Neurolinguistics (NLP)
A set of rather cult tools developed by an anthropologist and a CIA agent, Bandler and Grinder, have been translated into useful everyday language by a range of authors, notably Lankton and Cameron-Bandler. They are tools most applicable to demythologising drugs and drug use and can be most effective in changing behaviour or one's view of the world. Based on our principal strategies of taking in, storing and retrieving information through sight, sound or feelings, and the storing and accessing of that information by symbols, NLP is an appropriate tool to educate users on the symbolism their own drug holds for them.

Education as prevention

If we put education into the context of our framework for drug issues, we can see how effective and far-reaching educational strategies can be, given policy support and well-tried programs. We can also see the difficulties more clearly. A drug-educated teenager, with full knowledge of the options and the effects of drugs, may be hypercritical of drug-using parents and teachers, or may simply decide to copy them. Modelling is the single most powerful educational tool for humans. If educational strategies succeed in making individuals more self-reliant and responsible and more knowledgeable about their own community, then there is potential for conflict with the totem of teacher infallibility. If the avenues of control and treatment do not contain a preventive element, we have no potential for rehabilitation of imprisoned addicts, and the health care professions will continue to rearrange deck chairs on the *Titanic* as far as drug abusers are concerned.

The controversy over methadone provides a good example. If schools and higher education institutions distributed the information outlined in the previous chapter, with opportunity for discussion and understanding of the options, potential heroin users would not see methadone as an easy escape from addiction, nor would their friends (as happens today) aid and abet them in obtaining methadone in a way that they would not do to get them heroin. Health care providers who understand better the network of support needed for a methadone maintenance program would not leave all the support to the medical practitioners; and law enforcement staff would not see methadone as a simple control measure, but also co-operate with the rest of the support network.

In short, while education is perhaps our cheapest, most effective and longest lasting avenue of prevention, it is a toothless tiger without a supportive social context, and it must stem from a comprehensive policy which includes professional training for practitioners from all the avenues of approach to drug issues, the doctors, lawyers and police as well as the teachers themselves.

In using the holistic analysis of aspects of evidence, as we have done for the other strategies, in Table 23 we can see the strengths and weaknesses of this approach if it is forced to stand alone. Our hypercritical teenager may decide that education is hypocritical and try to avoid it altogether. While professionals in the treatment and control fields remain at such a distance from the realities of drug

EDUCATION   139

Table 23
Framework for drug issues 7: education as policy

	Avenues of approach			
	Control	Treatment	Education	Social change
Policy	The right to knowledge and understanding of drug use and abuse, in order to reduce abuse			
Aspects of strategy:				
Physical states	Learning physical symptoms of withdrawal; understanding results of constraint	Research into treatment results	Knowledge of human biology, including drug effects	Acceptance that the taboo exists, and can be studied
Ethical goals	Acceptance of use and abuse as human, not evil	Acceptance of use and abuse as the problems (not the person as the problem)	Acceptance of users and abusers as capable of learning	Acceptance of use and abuse as part of the human condition
Aesthetic responses	Reduce all risk taking; don't permit students to experience highs	Reduce physiological highs; call them hyperactivity and treat with drugs	Provide physiological highs by sport, competition	Recognition that aesthetic ('feeling great') needs must be met; should be channeled into socially acceptable forms
Social rules	Rehabilitation and education part of corrective services	Education as one component of treatment	Schools and colleges can discuss heroin use and abuse	Heroin users can declare themselves in need, without being either totem or taboo
Individual perspective (an ordinary citizen)	Need to know avenues for and success rates of, control	Need to know success rates of treatments	Need the young to explain *their* reasons for taking drugs	Education is totem, or socially acceptable path for community change in approach to drug use

issues, there is potential for conflict with the totem of professional infallibility. If education on drugs and their social context is extended to those fields as well as to schools, we have the beginning of the most effective educational tool of all—guided social change.

The participants in both the national Drug Summit and DA:NA gave the strongest support to education as the favoured preventive strategy, and to various avenues of social change as essential prerequisites to prevention. As we shall see in the following chapter, education and social change are inextricably linked.

9
Social Change

A prefigurative society

While education may be the preferred social option for prevention of drug abuse, social change is widely considered to be the most difficult and the most effective. Insofar as both are preventive measures, they stand and fall together. The first, however, fits most easily into our present social context; a situation which can be a problem as well as a strength when a teacher is working to change social values within a school. The second must, by definition, challenge existing social values and power structures, and can only succeed in the long run if linked with successful educational strategies and the overall consent of the community concerned. Since education is the path for socialisation of the young, change can only endure if the means of teaching the young are captured.

The sometimes confusing interactions between education and social change are clarified by the ways in which Margaret Mead describes three types of learning societies. She identifies the traditional society as one where all learning is transferred from the old to the young, which she calls postfigurative; in a changing society, young and old learn new ways together (cofigurative); and in the rapidly changing era of today, the new ways are so different from the old, that the young live in a world that the old cannot even recognise. In this last case, the young must teach the old, and Mead describes this as a prefigurative society, one in which the society is being re-shaped.

It is not difficult to draw analogies between drug use in Australia today and the third type of society. Drugs and their related customs move around the world with jet planes, global television, and mass transport; so that young drug cultures become ratified and unified, without the traditional need of support from their elders. The drug use itself becomes a totem to a group of young people who have no social identity: a flag of protest and 'the staff of life'. We badly need, therefore, effective strategies which reduce drug abuse in a way in which wedges are not driven between old and young, but which help each to learn from the other. Briefly, we need preventive measures which reach all groups of a society and help build, not destroy, its existing systems. Such measures will include education, in its broadest sense of the process of learning, since we will need means of dealing with social change that are non-disruptive. Community development strategies fit this last condition admirably.

Prevention has become a more popular option in recent years, for a number of reasons; not least because other methods have not succeeded in stopping abuse. Punishment and threat do not necessarily deter undesired behaviour. Preventive methods restricted to legislation against use of, or restricting access to, drugs are narrowly focused and ignore the reasons why people use drugs and persist in doing so despite formal opposition and despite risks to their health.

Other reasons for putting faith in community contributions to prevention are the growing awareness of the psycho-social and physical costs of abuse to individuals, families and society as a whole, and a belief that, logically, prevention of problems must be better than cure. It is also recognised that this approach has benefits for community well-being in general. But while community preventive action would appear to be an improvement on past methods it is not the cheap or easy solution it is often thought to be. Invoking this approach to prevention requires a serious, detailed analysis of what are the real problems and goals and a strong commitment to the solutions.

Community action

The classic parable of community action, for prevention of illness or promotion of health, is the ambulance story. Town dwellers, appalled by the number of suicides who made use of a local high cliff, clubbed together to buy an ambulance and build a road by which it could easily reach the foot of the cliff. After two years of the community's paying the running costs, with the number of suicides increasing, someone suggested building a fence at the top. Why didn't we think of that first, they said?

We don't think of prevention first. We think of more of the same, far more often than we think of changing our tactics. The following, perhaps daunting, list describes what is needed for a successful community intervention program.

Factors in success

Learning how the community works before intervening.

Remaining broad and multidisciplinary, co-ordinating many facets of information and resources.

Recognising that drug use is firmly entrenched in our society, that drugs are a source of pleasure and that they are unlikely to be eliminated.

Taking into account that behaviour has multiple complex causes which extend beyond individuals to the social and cultural environment in which they live.

Recognising that people need to be properly informed about the nature of drugs and motivated and enabled to abstain or to use them in non-abusive ways.

Understanding that people are already meeting their needs in the best way they know how.

Working with people to help them meet their needs as they see them, rather than imposing other's ideas on them.

Not working specifically with drugs and not expecting benefits to be confined to merely preventing drug abuse problems.

Not limiting responsibility to professionals or government agencies, but sharing it with individuals, families and communities.

Setting up ongoing, co-ordinated action plans, integrated into existing social structures.

Tailoring actions to meet the needs of high risk 'outsider' groups such as the children of alcoholics, unemployed teenagers and non-tribal Aborigines.

Working in concert with the strategies of education, treatment and control, linked in a series of interventions to have substantial impact.

Intervening on a number of fronts at once in the knowledge that the subject is complex, that different aspects need to be dealt with in different ways and that no single intervention can have the necessary impact.

Monitoring programs continually for wanted and unwanted effects. To do this successfully it is necessary to work from an information base on present patterns and the nature of drug use.

Evaluating by clearly specified goals, especially when the program involves nebulous factors such as self-esteem or community self-determination.

Empowering the community to nominate their own needs for change and to build them into their own society. If we don't, the whole effort will go for nought.

Avenues for success
Strategies for social change work through both individuals and the social environment. The individual approach recognises that people have needs which when not met in safe, acceptable ways are met in other less desirable ways—these include crime, delinquency or drug abuse. It takes into account personal choices of lifestyle, the moral and aesthetic choices the individual is free to make, and the social rules under which they are constrained. Attention must still be paid to the social environment of the individual because it determines the dimensions along which change is possible. Individuals particularly in need may well need rescuing first; working with key individuals can act as leaven in the social environment; either of these groups may need to be engaged before most of the population can be involved in a program.

Environmental strategies for social change to be effective must be carried out through the major institutions that already exist in our society, that is, the families, educational institutions, community groups, professions, work and social organisations, media, commerce and government. Together, such strategies can positively influence attitudes, behaviour and circumstances in ways which can decrease or inhibit the antecedents to drug abuse and the changes can be permanent because supported from within the community. Many authorities are pessimistic about the potential of established institutions for change, and quote a generation as the time needed for change to take place. These people cannot have observed the incredibly rapid changes in communication technology, in female sex roles, and in attitudes to the environment in the past decade.

Families

The family is the most obvious and immediate focus for intervening on an individual level, for it is there that the earliest socialisation occurs and children begin to develop self-images. The addict rehabilitation literature also reinforces the family's importance, with evidence that the majority of clients come from disturbed or broken families; particularly those where a parent lacked close involvement because of work, alcoholism or divorce.

This evidence draws attention to the need for parents to be better trained and equipped for their roles (both before and during parenting) and to be well resourced, both from the primary and secondary prevention angles, i.e. parenting needs to be included in school curricula and in courses for newly married people. They need to know of services such as parent support counselling, marriage guidance and child psychologists and also need encouragement to use them before their problems reach crisis point. Teachers and medical practitioners in particular need to be aware of early symptoms and of how best to encourage their contacts to seek help. It is worth noting that although some crisis centres exist, such as women's refuges, there is no respite care for parents with problems at the stage when they are still seen as minor. Such help would be particularly beneficial for those with no grandparents available. The totem of the self-sufficient family network still exists, long after the network itself is, not gone, but often no longer available as support.

Another problem is the generally prevailing attitude that it is unacceptable to admit to having problems. People need to be able to recognise when they are in need of outside help, and to re-examine their rules as to from whom and when it is permissible to ask for help. Parenting is no longer a 'natural gift' when most of us have now grown up in two-child families, in which we do not remember ever having seen a baby washed or fed. The social rules which will affect our children are different from those of our childhood. A prefigurative society indeed.

Parent self-help groups have proved useful and have the potential to be very effective, both for education and mutual support—and in some places they have been formed specifically to combat drug problems. The latter have provided parents with peer support to combat negative pressures that their children face from outside influences. Professionals have provided back-up assistance when required. However, it would appear that groups with an overall well-being approach have a better chance of being maintained and remaining problem free than those that arise to combat crisis abuse problems. The fence at the top of the hill is still more effective than the ambulance.

Social organisations

Involvement in cultural and sporting organisations can provide valuable socialising roles as well as opportunities for self-fulfilment, exploration, creativity and extension of abilities. They often promote physically healthy lifestyles and can distract from illegal or dangerous pastimes.

Sport in Australia is a dilemma to the prevention-oriented planner, however. On the one hand it appears to provide a useful avenue for healthy activities. The Australian Sports Medicine Foundation, for example, points out that participation in sport is one of the main reasons for abstinence from tobacco and alcohol among young people.

On the other hand, many popular sports promote competitiveness, are closely associated with an excessive macho image, including drinking and smoking, and separate sexes and age groups (and therefore divide families). It cannot be ignored that the image of Australia as a sporty nation is a myth because the majority do not exercise regularly and for each major sporting event there are few players and thousands of spectators. The Life. Be In It advertising campaign and set of community initiatives brought about a social change of consciousness, and the beginnings of a change in behaviour. Fun Runs, neighbourhood walks and Betsy's hoop were a great start; we must wait longer for the full evaluation.

For sport to positively promote mental and physical well-being, there needs to be a reassessment of the promoted activities. Men's sport needs to be dissociated from boozing, and the picture of the sporting hero as the epitome of health must be demystified.

Professional community development

One of the most interesting and potentially effective prevention interventions is that in which professionals assist a community to solve its own problems. This type of intervention has been operating in USA for twelve years and has recently been introduced to Australia by the Community Approach to Drug Abuse Prevention (CADAP) team (see Chapter 12).

CADAP focuses on the predisposing factors leading to drug abuse and related problems. Community members learn skills in problem analysis, action planning and implementation of programs which really meet the needs of their community. For example, in 1984 the CADAP team was invited to visit an isolated Northern Territory town to explain their approach. Some months later a team from the town went to Darwin for intensive training. The team included a dressmaker, school nurse, school counsellor, mining office worker, alcohol and drug counsellor and an educational psychologist (some of whom were parents).

The team identified a host of worrying features including few jobs and social activities, housing problems, lack of child care, parental absences because of shift work, shortage of older citizens and drug problems. Boredom was identified as the key issue and practical ways of dealing with it were devised. The different needs of youth, unemployed, mothers, single people and shift workers were taken into account. The team worked together on a public education program, school involvement program (from principals to primary school students), and a family fun day.

These are only the beginning of planned activities and illustrate what can be achieved by a concerned and active community with some initial specialised help.

Mass communication media

Modern media of mass communication influence the individual, but more importantly have a powerful role in influencing social

148 OUR DAILY FIX

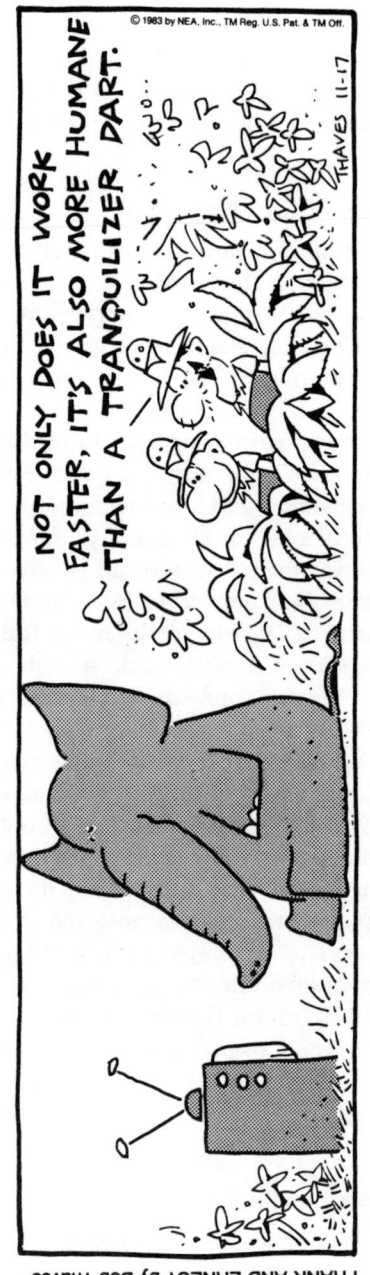

FRANK AND ERNEST by Bob Thaves

Cartoon by Thaves, reprinted by permission of United Press International on behalf of Newspaper Enterprise Association, from Australian, 14 November 1983 structure because of their ability to reflect, inform and publicise social trends and attitudes. To try and develop a successfully functioning community without acknowledging the power of the media would ignore one of the most potent influences in our society today.

To de-glamorise the drug topic and substitute accurate up-to-date information to assist rational public debate, the health professions need at least some members to establish and maintain close working relationships with the media. These need to recognise that skilled use of the media is an exacting social profession in itself and to work in co-operation with those who have such skills at their fingertips.

Some campaigns have been successful but most are ad hoc and research about them is sparse. The northern New South Wales Healthy Lifestyle Program of the late 1970s was one exception in that it was fully evaluated and reported (see Frape and Tyler). It is the responsibility of health educators to expand their knowledge about the media role, and to become equipped with specialist training in the area. The TV programs by Jonathan Miller on the BBC and *The body program* on Australian radio by Earle Hackett are cases in point, where medical educators have used electronic media as successfully as the most idolised current affairs program. TV in particular could be a most useful community tool if it extended its programs to cover subjects which educate, motivate and enable people to participate more fully in society; for example, programs on consumer rights showing people solving their own problems, descriptions of private and government agencies and the way that people can use them, parenting programs, descriptions of the activities and services of local clubs and societies. Some programs could serve particular groups, especially those at home during the day—retired people, mothers, the sick and unemployed. The content of these programs should be selected with input from viewing groups. Also the subtle but significant role that popular TV shows such as *A country practice* play should be valued and the shows examined for their message content about drugs.

Professional practices

Most health professionals are ill equipped to deal with the subject of drugs. Training at postgraduate and practitioner levels needs to be improved so health professionals recognise people with special needs, help people meet those needs in non drug-oriented ways if possible, appreciate the social context of people's problems and feel capable of helping people improve their situation. They need assistance to avoid the 'My doctor gives me pills to put him out of my misery' syndrome, as Wyndham said, or the even more insidious labelling of the person by their drug: 'that heroin addict is in the waiting room, doctor'.

In particular, doctors and pharmacists dispensing drugs need encouragement to counsel patients on the proper use of drugs, with particular attention given to prescriptions for paediatric and geriatric patients, and informing people about problems associated with alcoholic beverages. While it is comparatively simple, once the policy decision is made, to alter professional practice by altering the original degree program, it is infinitely more difficult to change the behaviour expected of practising professionals or to develop the skills of professionals to work in a team. Yet social change in the treatment of any drug abuse will depend, in the first instance, on presently practising professionals. The two strategies most needed are the ability to work in professional teams and a willingness to work with the client's family and social environment; both alien, as we discussed in the Treatment chapter, to the standard practice of private treatment today. FMECH (Foundation for Multi-disciplinary Education in Community Health) in Adelaide and the Newcastle Medical School explicitly train inter-professional teams, but this is rare elsewhere. SICH (Student Initiatives in Community Health) is nationally funded for the same purpose.

The other issue, the ability to work with clients' families and friends, is even more in conflict with the individualism of most professionals and indeed invades professional autonomy. Standards and confidentiality may be involved here. Standards for this type of professional practice have been thoroughly investigated by CHASP (Community Health Accreditation and Standards Project) mounted by the Australian Community Health Association, led by Denise Fry in New South Wales.

Advertising

Some control is already exerted over advertising but it needs to be increased in positive ways which do not necessarily alienate the commercial interests involved. It is considered by treatment agencies important to de-emphasise instant gratification and bought cures for problems and to dissociate popular social events from drug use, e.g. football and beer.

To be successful such efforts require influence, co-ordination and consistency and involve a number of levels of approach; for example, policy to have standards set and advertisements evaluated, legal enforcement of standards, workshops for commercial groups to assist them to recognise the significance of their role. Some of these approaches are already being taken, but their effectiveness is limited. Because of vested interests they lack real commitment. To be really successful the subject needs to be politicised much more strongly. The following is an excerpt from the NH&MRC Standing Committee on Health Promotion and Education's paper on 'The media and public health'.

> Advertising is big business. Australia is one of the most advertising-saturated societies in the world, ranking fourth in the world in terms of dollars per head of population spent on advertising. The tobacco industry spends approximately $60 million per annum promoting its products. Yet smoking is the second largest cause of death in Australia.
>
> Evidence suggests that the tobacco industry has actively engaged in countering health promotion campaigns. In the Lismore campaign in New South Wales, the tobacco industry placed substantial counter-advertising in the local press. During the campaign, advertising of tobacco products increased by at least 60 per cent on the previous year. During this same campaign, two companies complained to the Australian Media Council that the health advertisements disparaged their products. The health advertisements were temporarily withdrawn.
>
> The food industry provides yet another example of the relationship between advertising and health. Between 45 and 60 per cent of all advertising televised during children's 4 to 6 pm viewing time is for 'food' products which, a survey by the Australian Consumers' Association has found, are in direct conflict with the Commonwealth Department of Health's established priorities for health and nutrition education.
>
> The child who is called to the dinner table at six comes (on a fairly typical night) from watching three advertisements for ice treats, six for chocolates or chocolate-coated sweets, three for crisps snacks, one for a chocolate flavoured cereal, another for gum, and a couple of commercials for a fast food chain which likens meal time to a circus. Advertisements aim to develop an almost insatiable demand by children for such sugary rubbish and heavily salted fatty snacks.

The media contains hidden health agenda through the images it daily presents, particularly on television. Women see themselves as powerless. People with disabilities don't see themselves at all. You can't live in Marlboro country on a pair of crutches. Ethnic minorities are under- represented. This cannot but have a cumulative effect on concepts of identity and self-worth which are both essential elements in good health.

Feelings of guilt and inadequacy are regularly exploited in advertisements directed at women. For example, manufacturers of baby products show through their advertising that babies can be transformed from mewling and puking bundles of alarm to gurgling contented infants if they are only given the best bottled baby foods and the latest disposable nappies. Real life babies are not so easily fooled and the young inexperienced mother can be caught in a double bind. If she showers her infant with the latest of commodities and *still* the baby cries, she can feel both inadequate and alarmed. If she can't afford the products, she feels guilty.

The media therefore has the power and the potential to reinforce and prescribe social roles, and to perpetuate the disadvantage of certain social groups. Access to the media for the purpose of promoting health must not be confined to any one interest group but be open to a wide range of interested parties and be publicly accountable.

Social gathering places

Until recently, drug education programs have completely ignored the number one public source of (legal) drugs, that is, clubs and hotels. They might at first glance appear to be controversial places to intervene but experiences in Queensland have shown that this need not be so. The Queensland Hotel Patron Care Program trains hotel managers and bar attendants in responsible care of patrons who are beginning to abuse alcohol or have obvious problems. Not only does the service promote caring attitudes to the patrons and better attitudes to alcohol consumption, but it also improves behaviour and general atmosphere—which in turn encourages social drinkers and abstainers to patronise the facilities.

Pubs do not have to continue to be associated with 'boozing' to be financially viable. They could well extend their appeal to families, groups, older people and the young teenagers and regain their lost image as the social centre of the community.

Other popular gathering places such as shopping malls could examine how they could better meet the needs of those who 'hang out' there, usually with little money to spend in what is primarily a money-oriented place (e.g. youths, pensioners, and unemployed mothers). However, those involved in making profits are not usually concerned with providing cheap and stimulating activities in their expensive facilities and they may need persuading that they too have a role to play in making our social environment attractive and satisfying.

Work places

Because the majority of adults spend the major part of their non-sleeping lives at work, that environment is an important place on which to focus prevention activities. People are particularly accessible there and are often in groups which enable programs to be targeted to age, sex, ethnicity and education.

Work places need to be critically examined (by workers, unions and bosses) to determine whether the environment is conducive to mental and physical well-being. In some cases the remedies may be simple (e.g. adjusting shift times, or providing creches on-site), in some cases difficult (changing expensive equipment, or redesigning the building).

One outcome of effective prevention is that attitudes to drug use should change, becoming more responsible and non-blaming. A benefit of this change should be that people are more likely to report early symptoms or to accept help when their problems are detected by others (i.e. secondary prevention). The National Alcohol and Drug Dependence Industry Program is an example of a national program which works mainly at this secondary level. Both large and small industries and businesses are involved in the program which is organised by the Alcohol and Drug Foundation, Australia with Commonwealth assistance. It works by identifying problems in their early stages, as indicated by falling standards of work performances, and motivating people to seek assistance and promoting responsible attitudes to drug use in the work place.

There is much potential for developing this type of program, if the necessary back-up services can be provided.

Voluntary organisations

The strategies described above take account of Nowlis's statement that the greatest obstacle to understanding and responding to behaviour involving drugs is the belief that, because a drug is involved, the behaviour is unique and requires new research, specially trained experts, new and special methods of intervention and treatment.

In any functioning community we already have many of the necessary structures to carry out an effective ongoing program of prevention. By definition a community is a self-supporting group of people. The real problem may not be a lack of resources but rather a lack of co-ordination, direction and knowledge. The impetus for real, concerted action lies not with governments or professionals but with individuals and community groups.

Once we have a policy commitment to community development, the next step is to resource and empower the members of that community to work well with established social structures, and to contribute to the social change. Their great advantage is a grass roots familiarity with the issues, and a capacity for immediate action. Community members do not need to wait for money, bureaucratic permission, or scientific proof of need. Margaret Mead's third type of society, the prefigurative, cannot survive without making use of these strengths.

In *Don't mourn for me—organise*, David Scott lists five aspects of social reform, in all of which voluntary groups are crucial. First, as experimenters and innovators: most of the current welfare services have been pioneered by voluntary groups and organisations, for instance family planning, community health centres and outreach hospital services. Second, volunteers are free to undertake work labelled as revolting and/or unnecessary by the paid worker. The example of Mother Teresa picking up the dying from the streets of Calcutta dramatises what goes on in neighbourhoods every day: the care of someone else's incontinent parent or the availability of a homebound neighbour for lonely children. Third, public welfare services would be impossibly expensive if not linked to complementary voluntary services. Fourth, agencies tend to drift away from servicing the clients' needs towards an orientation to the needs of the providing professional, unless kept in touch by a well-organised client group. Schon's case study of the Blind Society in the 1950s illustrates this point. The workers of that Society kept Blind Institutes comfortable places in which the inmates remained blind; yet modern technology was available which could allow them to move about freely. Fifth, in the increasingly impersonal world of big cities and big government, voluntary organisations provide opportunities for personal services and friendship, for self-fulfilment, and for worthwhile contributions from people who are not otherwise valued within their social context.

Two further potential roles for volunteer workers are predicted by Scott. There is the need to take back some of the roles abrogated without realising it to institutions and professions; examples of this are the movement of some parents to take over at least some of the teaching of their children themselves, the home birth movement, and bereavement counselling groups. The other potential community role is the need for voluntary work by the powerful on behalf of the disempowered; the nineteenth century gives us graphic illustrations of this, as in Wilberforce and the slave trade.

In Australia, such groups are already working for Aboriginal land rights, single parents and intellectually handicapped children. The need for similar groups to work with and on behalf of the drug addicted is clear, as the Richmond Fellowship and Odyssey House have shown us already.

Self-help groups

Self-help groups are another vitally important medium of modern social change. Scott, who has spent thirty years promoting and empowering such groups, mostly in Melbourne with the Brotherhood of St Laurence but also in India with Community Aid Abroad, points out that it is accepted that self-help groups of the powerful self-interested run the country; these are the business, farmer, union and professional lobbies which can bargain with their money, goods, labour or services.

Disadvantaged or outsider groups need to discover their own internal strategies and external bargaining power. For the drug impaired or drug dependent, involvement not only improves confidence, enhances skills and gives a sense of purpose (all likely to reduce the grip of the drug) but it brings an awareness of the power systems of the local community and lessens the feelings of helplessness and victimisation by fate, typical of case studies of drug users. For those condemned to isolation by the conspiracy of silence, or taboos, of overuse of legal drugs or any use at all of illegal drugs (the wife of the alcoholic or the parent of the heroin user) a self-help group is often the only avenue of escape for themselves or their family. ACA (Adults, Children of Alcoholics) groups are examples of this, a recent much-needed initiative.

Self-help groups, to function effectively, need skill in the following areas: negotiation and lobbying, identification of targets, planning implementation and evaluation of a strategy, use of the media, personal and group problem solving, crisis resolution, team building and learning access to resources. Any drug strategy which supplies those skills to a group abusing drugs, or a group at risk of abuse, will clearly need courage and perseverance in the short term, but there are plenty of dramatic long-term examples of success: Alcoholics Anonymous, women's and youth refuges.

Consumer organisations

Consumer groups are a special form of self-help group with a powerful part to play. Consumer groups in the area of drug abuse may sound a little unrealistic, not to say antisocial, but consumer groups for any of the strategies which respond to drug abuse are an essential component of the success of the strategy. Health care groups in Canberra and in Sydney have helped redesign the health care systems of their communities. Clarification of clients' rights and responsibilities allows a dignified interaction between providers and receivers of care, and acts as a built-in brake to errors of judgment on either side. Canberra Consumers Inc. distribute a pamphlet, legally accurate, but written in everyday language, on the rights and responsibilities of the consumer in the health field.

In two particular ways, consumer groups are an essential component of social change: (a) as the young or the disadvantaged they are 'the other side of the coin' needed to re-educate members of established society to a changing world, and (b) they, and only they, can truly evaluate the services delivered as successful or unsuccessful strategies. The flood of books on the powerlessness of the client and patient (Taylor, Szasz) and the changes in client-professional relationships attest to a generation of professional care givers which forgot to listen to its consumers.

In Australia, while we have only a few localised health care consumer groups we have many general consumer groups and two strong centralised groups: Australian Consumers' Association (ACA), based in Sydney, publishes *Choice*, whose sales fund excellent consumer research; and Australian Federation of Consumer Organisations (AFCO), based in Canberra, which has representation on many national policy bodies, including the National Health and Medical Research Council and its constituent committees. Consumers are not powerless; neither are they only concerned with products and services bought and paid for. We are all recipients of many services whether we like it or not. How the law is administered, when penalties for cannabis use vary from a caution in one city to a year's gaol in another; neglect of and contempt for elderly alcoholics in casualty departments of major hospitals, and over-medication of hospital inpatients, are all consumer concerns. Often unable to speak in the language of the care providers, consumers need a platform or a spokesperson. To call into question totems, such as search techniques of the police drug squad, or taboos, such as medical practitioners whose practice is entirely adolescents on 'uppers' and 'downers', needs support from the community. Consumer groups provide that support.

Search conferences

Springing from an idea germinated in Australia, future-oriented planning groups have developed into a worldwide phenomenon for rethinking policy, strategy or direct action. Fred and Merrelyn Emery have published widely the results of their strategy of looking fair and square at social change and its consequences for any service area or client group. Taking sufficient time (one day to two weeks) away from base, incorporating the concerned group and the community network (for instance, a university psychology course, its students and the potential employers in the community), rethinking the issues from the ground up, and ending with concrete steps all wish to take, search conferences have helped many long-established institutions change gear. The skilled group leader from outside the area and the time detached from everyday concerns are essential ingredients in their success.

Negotiating skills

Search conferences as a social phenomenon reveal how much western society is conscious of the need to rethink priorities. The flood of courses and books on negotiating skills reveals how universal is the threat of conflict and deadlock in western society at present. Social change, as we have discussed, carries with it the threat of disruption, of loss of power to the powerful, of loss of skill to the skilled. Some confidence that matters will be thoroughly explored and argued about is a vital element in the security of both the powerful and the powerless. While search conferences provide a terrain where this can be done in a creative way, negotiating skills are needed in day-to-day conditions of change.

Fisher and Ury of the Harvard project have produced a useful set of guidelines in *Getting to yes*. They use a three-step process. First, isolating the issue from the position (as for example in separating the issue of the boredom of unemployment from the attitude which condemns unemployed youth as drop-outs and magic mushroom eaters). Second, finding the potential for agreement within the areas of disagreement (as in reconciling 'we all care about our children' with 'kids without jobs are drop-outs'). Third, taking the concrete steps for solution from the theoretical arguments (offer the group who are into magic mushrooms a chance to train for a job). The three steps can be seen as the keys to successful problem solving.

Non-violent action

Another avenue to resolving the potential for conflict inherent in social change is the technique of non-violent action. Community groups have used such techniques (well summarised in a three-volume work by Sharpe) to alert the rest of their society to important issues. BUGA-UP (Billboard Utilising Graffitists Against Unhealthy Promotions) is a group who feel strongly about smoking. Their exploits of 'refacing' giant hoardings which advertised tobacco used the might of the advertising agency against itself. After several years of changing 'Marlboro Country' to 'Cancer Country', BUGA-UP members when arrested for defacing the billboards successfully argued in court that their work was in the public interest. The campaign diverted the advertising agencies' use of totem and taboo to sell products to that of reducing their use. Then the effective defence of their case, argued in the centre of the control mechanisms which enforce the law, showed the strength of direct action in negotiating changes in community attitudes.

Social change revisited

Social change sounds a dramatic, not to say draconian, answer to a national problem. But due consideration allows us to identify (a) that we live in an era of acute social change, so that we may as well learn to direct it where we would like it to go; (b) drug use is often a symptom of reactions to existing social change, so that an understanding of the mechanisms of social change is necessary in order to understand drug abuse; and (c) human societies are essentially tools of social change since the overriding characteristic of human beings is not only the ability to learn but the inevitability that they will learn, and so change their society.

The same framework for drug issues we have used for an overview of the drug problem (Table 2), to look at specific drug use (Table 3), and to consider the implications of policy (Table 7), we now use to pinpoint appropriate prevention strategies. The implications for policy and social context are considerable, since social change calls existing rules into question. Table 24 contains a summary of the important points which need to be considered here, and which would accompany any serious move to prevent drug abuse.

The first point to note is that a fully preventive strategy has repercussions for all avenues of approach and response. Control and treatment are usually exercised after the event, and education in its formal sense has a full set of subjects which reinforce the knowledge rules of the day. These rules are included in the training of lawyers and the health care professions. A change to prevention, when that is a serious, comprehensive policy change, *is* social change, in that the social context must be altered to accommodate the necessary changes in existing totems and taboos.

We have discussed the power of the community itself when change is needed; but to encourage community responsibility is to reduce the power of the totem professions, law, medicine and

Figure 7   Alcohol in the headlines (see over)

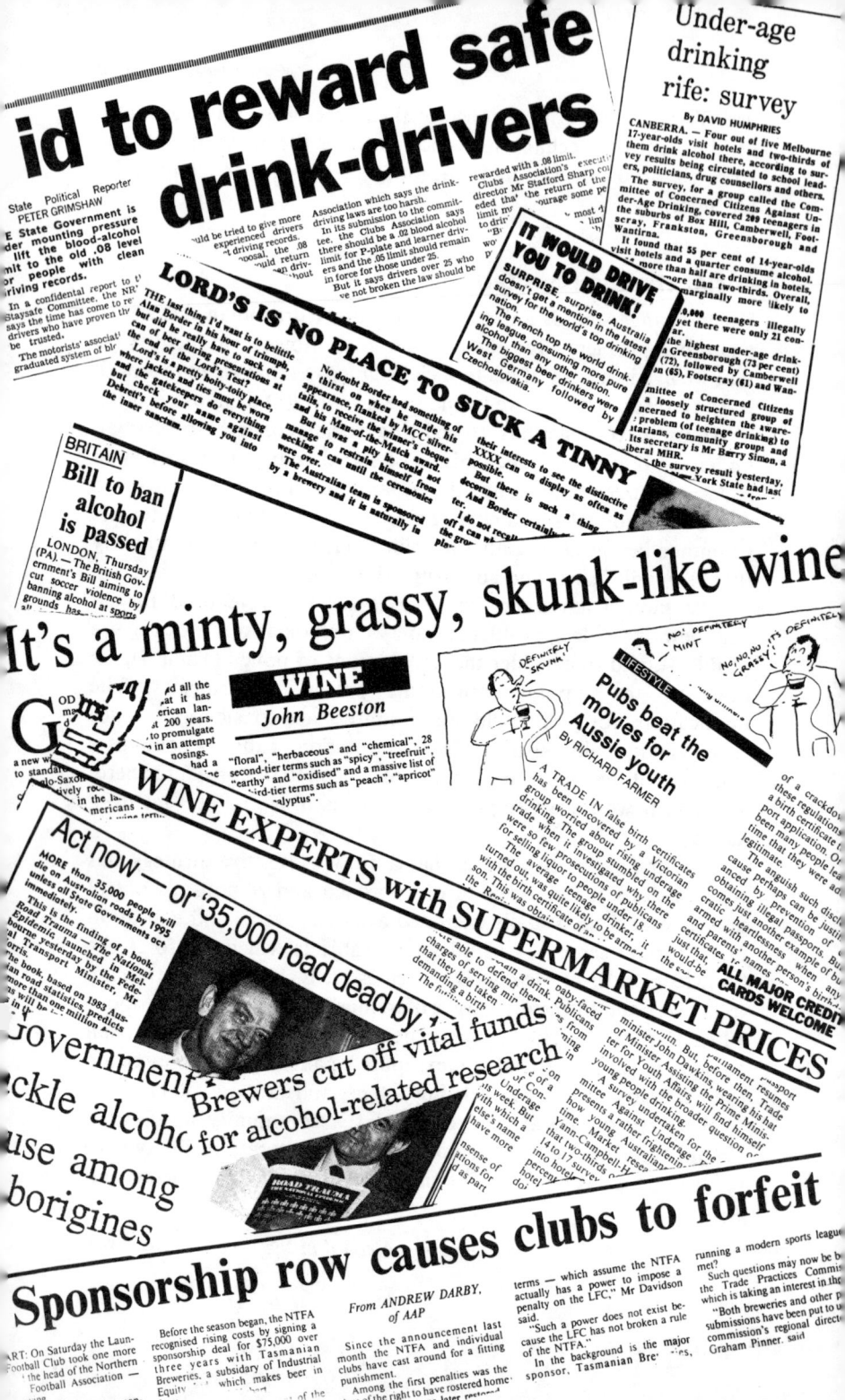

Table 24
Framework for drug issues 8: prevention as policy

	Avenues of approach and response			
	Control	Treatment	Education	Social change
Policy	Prevention is better than cure			
Social context (at present)	Seen as protective, powerful, necessary; conflicts with a high value for individual rights.	Seen as curative, specialised, authoritative.	Seen as a grounding in specialised content and skills, and in learning social rules.	Seen as 'only face problems after they arise'; disruptive, uncomfortable, unnecessary.
Strategy (for change)	Reduce availability of abused substances. Control abusers for treatment purposes.	Consider problems of origin of drug use (as well as consequences). Use patient education as one arm of treatment.	Broaden curriculum to include self-development, political skills, social competences. Analyse social totems and taboos. Interpret drug use.	Raise community consciousness of issues. Mobilise resources. Identify social networks. Identify interest groups.
Action	Change legislation; in-service programs for lawyers. Change police training methods.	In-service programs. Change professional training and research priorities.	In-service programs. Include self-esteem, self-assertion, body owner programs in formal education. Accept life-long education. Let the elders learn from the young.	(a) Search conferences (b) Train the trainer (c) Implement action plans across the board (d) Evaluate

education. Self-help groups of addicts can be seen as a contradiction in terms; just as self-help groups outside institutions for sufferers from schizophrenia were initially rejected as a danger to society and so taboo. Probably the only way to ensure that social change actually does occur is to take Mead's advice and make sure that the young are advising the old, and that young ideas and innovations are given space in all avenues of approach and response. This calls into question yet another totem. What we may need, most of all, are new totems and new taboos to underline the changes in drug use we wish to make and establish them within the social framework.

Such changes would take a national political initiative supported by the national will.

PART 3

ACTION:
Balancing Drug Use and Abuse

10
Changing The World

The third step

Action on a drug issue demands three steps: policy statement, strategy choice and direct action. The three steps are the same, whether the action is an arrest, detoxification, or taking a school class. The first two steps, as we have seen in Parts 1 and 2, are difficult enough, but the third puts the whole enterprise to the test. And it is not even as if the results of the action are always clear, or that the community concerned will always welcome it.

To change our world with regard to drug use and abuse is not an easy task, and many would ask, why should we try? The answer is that society has superimposed such a confusing system of values and counter-values upon the whole issue of drug use that it is impossible to seriously consider any reduction of abuse which deals with the drug alone. The scope of the subjects conveyed by that four-letter word 'drug' is vast, the uses are almost infinitely varied, and the reasons for abuse complex. The social context in which the drug taking is condemned or condoned, prescribed or proscribed is a vital element in an understanding of what the drug problem is about. Those who have not considered this perspective on drug taking will almost certainly fail to appreciate the entrenched position of drugs in society—and indeed in their own lives.

What the public sees, and the consumer of drug preventive services experiences, is yet another potential area for divergent views, when contemplating action. The detoxification units, schools, and remand centres are staffed by dedicated men and women, but the gulf between their best intentions, their clients' views of their own best interests, and the public's opinions of a proper policy can be wide indeed.

The diagram presented as Figure 1 is not intended to suggest that the path from policy to strategy to action is to be taken for one avenue of approach at a time, although this is sometimes the unspoken assumption. For a truly successful approach to drug problems, trains of thought, such as policy and social context, as well as trains of events, such as strategy and direct action, must be flexible, utilising all the different avenues. The more the artificial distinctions between doctors, lawyers, indians and chiefs can be broken down, so that everyone can see all of the options, the better.

The reader, in deciding where he or she stands on particular drug issues (such as legalisation of cannabis or the prohibition of brewery sponsorship of sport), must do a great deal more than consider facts and figures. Such empirical aspects are only one part of the evidence. We need to distinguish the ethical goals hidden in most broad policy questions, such as 'to what extent are we justified in restricting drug use which injures only the user?' In considering the cause of hard-drug abuse, it is important to consider the aesthetic and social value placed on the happy nuclear family and hence the effect that marital breakdown may have in creating a feeling of self-blame, and low self-worth among parents and children alike: exactly the preconditions for drug abuse. Strategies can be decided on in theory, but actions can only be chosen after we know what is the substance of abuse. There is certainly a policy against children's use of drugs, and strategies, such as curtailing access to drugs, which support the policy. But what is the action being taken on children buying the new bagged form of nicotine to suck? And a company which sells school supplies is selling skin stickers for children which can be scratched to release the smell of beer, martini or new money. Is action needed on this?

If we agree that there are not only the sixteen points, created by cross-referencing avenues of approach to drug use and levels of action, but a third dimension of four aspects of evidence to be considered, we have a three-dimensional world, with the points to be considered rising to sixty-four. Such a notional cube reflects the complexity of reality, and so is a more realistic, if more challenging, approach than a unidimensional view. We have not suggested, however, that people discard the coloured spectacles which give them their own particular world view. Rather, we have stressed that it is important to identify the colour of the glass, and to respect the coloured lenses of others. For understanding drug use and reducing abuse, all colours of the spectrum are required. Eventually we might reach white light and see clearly.

We expect those reading this book to cast a critical eye over our handiwork, too. We must practise what we are preaching. Perhaps we have allowed a penchant for analogy and metaphor to cloud the real picture of physical and emotional agony connected with drug abusers. But we have very much wanted to provide a learning tool, so that people can consider the analogy, or apply the metaphor, whatever the drug in question. But as we have noted, the step to action takes us into the real world, and for that we need evidence on which to act.

Acting on the evidence

We now know enough about drug use to interpret its role in society. All drugs taken for non-biological or non-therapeutic reasons contribute to a change of consciousness in some way; any society condones some methods of altering consciousness and condemns others. In Table 8 we saw that effects of drug taking can be euphoria, stimulation or relaxation. Since these are all highly sought after aspects of the human condition, and socially encouraged in other ways, when we act to reduce drug use we can be labelled killjoy, wowser, reactionary or bigot. When the drug being used is the basis of commercial empires, then one is at risk of further social criticism, not to say character assassination. Even when it is agreed that the chemical concerned is being abused, the activist in the field is rarely hailed as hero or heroine, as they might be if they tackled leprosy or cot death. Workers are more likely to be seen to be involved in a dirty business, and defiled by the taboos which accompany illicit drugs. We have heard how treatment of drug abuse is poorly funded, lacking adequate research, and a difficult area in which to recruit staff. In education, neither drugs nor even basic human biology have a respected place in the school curriculum. It is not much consolation that neither do driving or vocational skills, two other most necessary skills in real life.

Nothing succeeds like success, however, and perhaps the low morale described for workers in the drug abuse field is due, as well as to a sense of trying to beat back the tide, to an inability to show success when it has been achieved. This difficulty can be traced, in turn, to the paradoxes which bedevil action in that field. Although social change has been identified as a preferred option for prevention of drug abuse in our review of the situation in Part 2, we were left with two contradictions: first it is not possible to define a clear line between use and abuse, and so it is not at all clear when one should act; and second, it is unrealistic to expect to stop use and intolerable to live with a high level of abuse.

These dilemmas are nicely illustrated, and indeed clarified, by the proposition put to the Minister for Health, Dr Blewett, by the Alcohol and Drug Foundation, Australia, and subsequently read by him to the National Summit on drug abuse:

> There is no doubt that those substances of dependence which have the greatest per capita consumption cause the greatest damage to the physical, mental and social well-being of the community. However, some illicit drugs of dependence which have a very much smaller per capita consumption cause social problems out of proportion to their consumption through the impact on law and order because of graft, corruption, violence, robbery, etc. In the first of these areas moderating demand and in the latter reducing demand to a minimum should be given the highest priority.

The desired social change must be, therefore, to balance use and abuse, and this we know must invoke ethical goals, social rules, the aesthetic senses, and the range of individual perspectives in a community. It would seem from the evidence that such a balance is gradually becoming more ethically acceptable and socially permissible. Prohibition of alcohol failed, total rejection of drugs such as LSD has succeeded and prohibition of heroin has failed; for the second, because the drug cultures themselves rejected LSD, for the third, because heroin is fulfilling a social purpose for at least some members of society. Discussion still rages over marijuana, and alcohol, but agreement has been reached that marijuana use (although illicit) should not be a criminal offence which mars the user for life, and that alcohol (although licit) is the most widely abused drug, and the abusers need help. A balance is dimly emerging.

There is recognition of the need for a policy which seeks a balance, rather than a cut-off point, between the use and abuse of any one drug, a community readiness to examine a social change as an avenue of prevention, and acceptance of the value of all avenues of approach being invoked in any adequate strategy. In Part 2 we proposed a scheme which involves all five aspects of evidence in developing the appropriate strategies for action. What more do we need?

That firm basis on which to take the third step.

Judging the outcome

It is one thing to look at past societies and identify the social uses of the prevailing drugs, with their place as totem or taboo (as in Chapter 2), or to review the political options (as we did in Chapter 3), and even to have available all the evidence of physical effects and statistical evidence of use (as we present in Chapter 4). It is yet another to change any of those things. After we have selected our favoured strategy, choosing programs which are not only consistent with policy but which will implement the selected strategy and which we believe will work in practice, we have come half-way. We can still only succeed if workers in this uncertain field are prepared to evaluate their interventions and programs, so that the rest of us, who come after, can be more effective.

McLuhan has written of a changing society as a whirling wheel, where to cling to the edge is to be involved in the fastest change; but if people wish a perspective they must move to the centre, where the momentum is less and one can see what is going on. The trouble is that it is both scary and risky to let go the edge and move to the centre and no one is more aware of this than those at the 'whirling edge' of drug abuse services. Doing the best they can, it can seem irresponsible to take time out for theoretical considerations, and a personal affront to suggest an evaluation of those services, which usually depend on a highly dedicated staff, working under adverse conditions. But if one accepts the responsibility of changing the world then one must do it properly, and moreover one must know what one is doing.

To evaluate a community initiative we need a method which, far from ignoring all these aspects of the evidence, takes account of them. This would allow the interested parties to make their judgments on matters which they can understand. Such an effort asks for a prior acceptance that the matter in hand is complex, important and difficult to resolve. Drug use in Australia would seem to be such an issue and the initiation of a national campaign would appear to confirm the importance.

In describing the aims, practice and effect of an intervention, we need a method of evaluation which can take account of the complexities of social rules, the abstractions of moral positions, the intangibles of aesthetic choices, and the wide range of apparently incompatible positions among those involved, and at the same time be based on the sound scientific methods which brought such success to physical medicine. Just as important, we need evaluation methods which are sensitive to the needs of the service provider and the client; and the evaluation instrument must enhance, and not inhibit, the goals of a program. In physical science it is now accepted that the mere use of a measuring instrument will affect the conditions being measured; how much truer this is of a sensitive treatment or education program. A survey of consumers conducted halfway through painful withdrawals from Valium could well stop a program in its tracks; a study of a rehabilitation community may well shatter the illusions of a religious group who was funding it, show a high recovery rate, and yet record a high rate of 'burn out' of staff. Is this success? On whose terms? We need answers to such questions.

In Chapter 5, we suggested that any successful strategy in the prevention of drug abuse would have to act on five dimensions at once. Collecting evidence on all of those five aspects of a program also gives us the basis for the holistic evaluation we are seeking. The following aspects of the evidence need to be collected.

(a) *Physical:* the statements of objectives; the resources available; the behaviours of the planning committee, the secretariat, the participants and the target audience; the match between the stated objectives and the outcome; records of intended and unintended outcomes; the differential effects of drugs, and the conditions in which they are used.

(b) *Ethical:* the purpose, the values, the ideolgical positions and the moral perspectives of those involved. All of these affect the potential for success and the interpretation of the outcomes. There can be several sets of conflicting ethical positions in one program.

(c) *Aesthetic:* the standards of taste, fit, and effectiveness which guide those who set the objectives, the executors of the plans, and the interpreters of the outcome. Does the program 'feel' right? If it doesn't, it won't work or if it does work, it won't last.

(d) *Social:* the rules, the norms, the conduct for those involved, which limit and condition both objectives and outcomes. This includes the political set and the cultural constraints in which the intervention takes place. Social rules may be in conflict with each other when totems are being questioned.

(e) *Individual:* the position of the individual in the intervention. Since there is no such person as 'the normal' or 'the ideal' human being, knowledge of the range of individuals involved in a community initiative is essential. The way in which those individuals view their own position is crucial to the success of the intervention. Assumptions, expectations and prejudices are to be stated explicitly and collected as evidence rather than ignored. The assumptions and expectations of the observers need equally to be stated, and not concealed.

These five aspects of the evidence are certainly not mutually independent. The empirical evidence, that is, the physical observations and measurements, cannot be interpreted without knowledge of the ethical, aesthetic and social assumptions made by and about the group involved. The range of individual positions in the group is at least as important as estimating the average or the norm, because this range gives the potential for change. Each individual in turn will hold an ethical, a social and an aesthetic position on any issue, and none of the positions can be studied without empirical observations of behaviour.

For example, one could evaluate the program to reduce foetal damage resulting from pregnant heroin addicts (an actual program of the Bourke St Drug Advisory Centre). The program, now known as Phoebe House, puts pregnant heroin addicts on methadone maintenance and seeks to prevent the newborn child from enduring heroin withdrawal. Physical evidence would include physical effects of heroin and methadone on mother, foetus and subsequent child; the behaviours which link mother and child; the physical status of addiction of each six, twelve, and twenty-four months later; the physical diagnostics of health (energy balance, stress symptoms, diet, and life events) at the same stages of withdrawal; and the expectations as stated by professionals, peers and the mother at those stages. That empirical evidence would be of little use without cross-reference to the following:

(a) *The purpose of the parent of entering the program:* an ethical conviction about the responsibility of a parent; social pressures not to endanger a child; or an aesthetic choice that an addicted newborn is repulsive?

(b) *The goals of the program:* the welfare of the mother; the welfare of the child; an aesthetic conviction that methadone addiction is preferable to heroin addiction; social pressures to protect the newborn even at the expense of the parent; or a personal desire to test a theory?

(c) *The expectations of the funding agency:* is it an ethical imperative that both mother and child return to society unaddicted, or is the aesthetic of an addicted child again paramount; does the reputation of the agency need a successful intervention, or is the personality of the agency leader that of a risk taker?

Five-sided evaluation

This five-sided approach to evaluation takes the form of a wheel or a pentagon of five linked processes rather than the five levels implied by Tables 17, 18, 21-23. The five-dimensional approach is more accurately represented in Figure 8, where it can be further seen that the five components of the evaluation should each be collected in turn from three groups of players in the game, that is, the three levels of people who will influence events (policy makers, strategists and clients). At the centre is the observer, or team of observers, who in the end will have to make a complete story out of the evidence so collected.

Use of the first four criteria (physical, ethical, aesthetic and social) provides accuracy and reliability. The individual dimension provides an evaluation with sophistication and political reality, and allows consideration of the range of interest groups involved: the powerful, the powerless, the traditional, the radical, the old and the young. All groups have their own ethical goals, social rules and aesthetic choices, based on their empirical experiences in the real world. The recognition of the five dimensions permits consideration of the implicit and explicit aspects of the enterprise, and links the quantitative factors to the qualitative aspects.

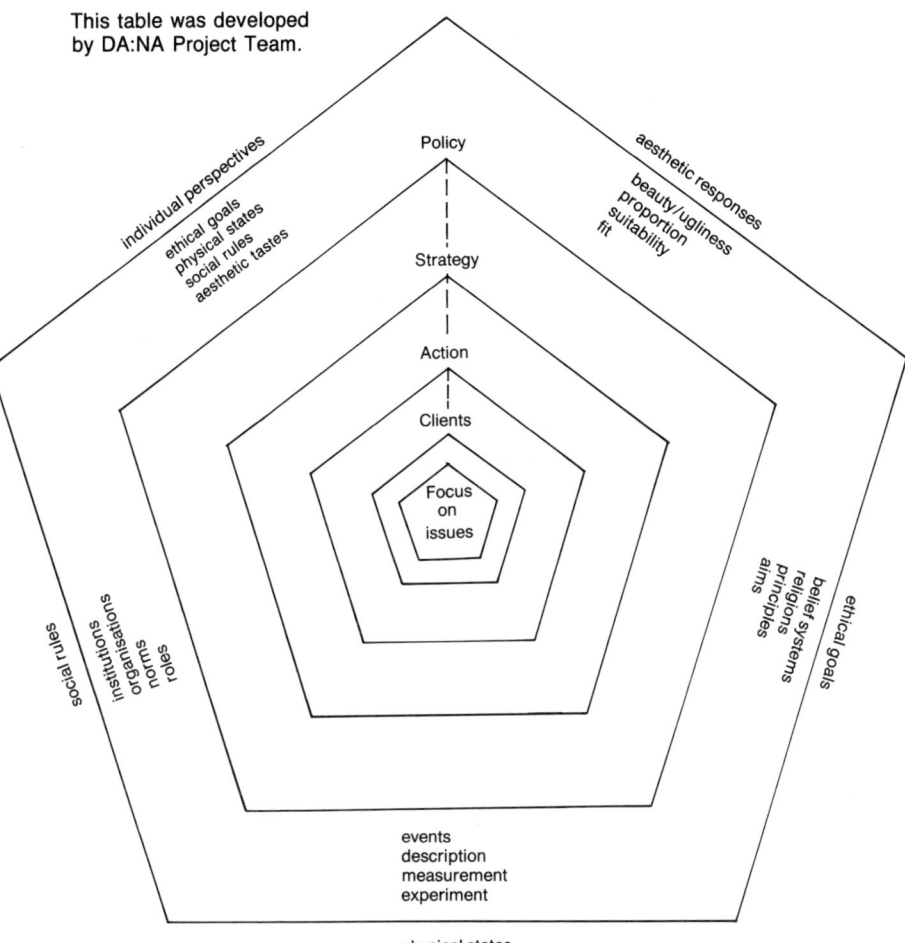

Figure 8 Evaluating the action : a five-sided approach

Before and after measures

The judgment of success must be related not only to what was intended (the aims and objectives of those concerned), but also to what one started with. To know how far one has come one needs a benchmark. Thus, a measure of the status quo is an essential beginning for an evaluation.

To satisfy stringent scientific requirements, each individual or society in this way will provide its own control. The change in any individual has its own validity; if that individual is typical, has leadership qualities, or is a social isolate, the changes in behaviour have different implications for the group.

Before and after measures are the stuff of scientific measurement. The level of addiction, the groups addicted, the recovery rates, the choice of drug, the social effects of the use of each drug, all provide the benchmarks needed for prediction of the effect of an intervention.

As well as before and after measures, there is a need to consider not only the explicitly stated but the implicitly assumed. There is also the expected and the unexpected, the wanted and unwanted, and the events compatible and incompatible with our original objectives. An evaluation to be useful is a full descriptive record of what happened, not a black and white judgment.

Such a multifaceted evaluation may be conceivable for single programs such as Phoebe House for pregnant heroin users, or to explain the dilemmas and paradoxes surrounding the individual addict, but is it robust enough to evaluate a complex set of programs, or the overall results of a policy decision? We can but try.

We have at our disposal evidence on the events leading up to a National Campaign Against Drug Abuse and descriptions of the programs available in Australia at the time. A five-dimensional analysis of this evidence provides a benchmark for evaluation of the success of the Campaign.

11
A National Campaign Against Drug Abuse

A national initiative

We have been considering the issues involved in changing the world —changing the world, not in this instance for a generalised Utopia, but to eliminate a known social canker. The social intricacies of drug use, the ineptness of policy formulation in the area, and the complexity of the conditions needed to influence social change could well make the strongest quail at attempting the task. Changing the world may well seem not only impossible, but one only the drug-affected would try. It may help for us to analyse one current Australian initiative for social change; one which holds a good set of cards, in that there are many factors to promote success.

The Prime Minister described in the opening paragraphs of Chapter 1 had himself come to power after overcoming acute addiction to alcohol. Having made an election promise that there would be an effective national campaign against drug abuse, starting with a conference between himself and the Premiers of the States and Territories, he allocated $60 million over three years to reducing drug abuse in Australia. This strong commitment from the top meets one condition that Schein predicted as necessary for social change: someone in power with an intention to achieve the change. In Chapter 12 we will review Schein's other prerequisite: people at the grass roots who can bring it about.

In the National Campaign, announced the Prime Minister:

> there will be emphasis on educating Australian youth about the damage and danger of drugs, and on rehabilitation of those in our society with

drug-related problems. Action on these points will complement the Commonwealth's commitment to enforce and to tighten the laws relating to drug offences.

Thus all four strategies for reducing drug abuse were to be called into play, and if the high level of representation at the Summit is any guide, serious consideration was to be given to policy. Given this encouraging start, we can proceed to set up the pentagon system of evaluation for the National Campaign. For this, we need a broad range of evidence by which to establish the objectives various groups expect the Campaign to fulfil, and from these objectives we can derive the criteria against which the Campaign can be judged.

Sources of evidence of aims and objectives are: political statements, workshop recommendations, submissions from the public, media coverage, statistics on extent of drug use, pharmacology of drug effects. From the last two, we can expect to estimate physical limits, and from the first two the ethical goals by which the community judges abuse. From the middle two we should be able to identify some of the social rules being applied to drug use and abuse, and the range of opinion on, not only those rules, but standards of permissiveness and taste. Fortunately for this enterprise, in the short four months from announcement of the National Campaign to Summit the amount of material produced was immense.

For our present purpose, we will take excerpts from politicians' speeches to DA:NA and the Prime Minister's announcement of the Campaign as our sample of political opinion; although, in this case, it is certainly a biased sample, of politicians with a special concern for the community. Statistics and pharmacology we have reviewed in Chapter 4. Now we will look in detail at the design and outcomes of workshops held to advise the Summit of community views, the submissions from the general public and the interpretations in the daily press.

A national community drug workshop

On 3 January 1985, a committee of nine (as listed in the Preface) met to initiate plans for a national drug workshop which was to advise the Summit meeting of Prime Minister and Premiers. The title of the workshop was to be Drugs in Australia: National

Action, with the acronym DA:NA. After three extensive meetings the aim and objectives of the workshop were established as follows:

Aim

To contribute to the formulation of strategic policies at the Special Conference of Premiers for a National Campaign Against Drug Abuse as outlined in the Prime Minister's press statement of 20 December 1984, in which education of youth and rehabilitation of those affected by drug- related problems were emphasised.

Objectives

1. To obtain an informed community view of the nature and extent of the drug problem in Australia.
2. To provide a critical approach to the information available to allow the community to make a balanced assessment of the 'drug problem'.
3. To examine what kind of relationship to drugs we believe desirable for Australian citizens and the society we want.
4. To decide whether governments are justified in enacting legislation which will significantly limit existing civil liberties in attempting to control the supply and distribution and use of certain drugs.
5. To determine whether drug abuse should be formally accepted by governments as a national public health problem rather than an issue of law and order.
6. To evaluate the need for over-riding national policies and co-ordinated legislation. For example, a similar approach to the postwar national tuberculosis campaign.

It was agreed that recommendations were needed on the following:

Methadone program
Registration of drug addicts
Supply of heroin to addicts
Recognition of alcohol and tobacco as major contributors to health and social problems
The inter-relationship of all drug use
A centre of international standing for drug and alcohol studies
Enforced treatment: diversion from the legal system to medical care
Legalisation or decriminalisation of marijuana use

Treatment programs within corrective services
The place of the media in controlling abuse
Advertising of socially approved drugs
Professional training
Reducing criminal profits
Confiscation of property
Who foots the bill?
Database requirements.

The Committee also developed the range of moral and social questions listed at the close of Chapter 1.

Workshop design
Prior to the workshop the participants received (a) a telex from the Prime Minister, (b) a personal invitation from the Minister for Health and (c) a letter from the Organising Committee asking for their involvement with the content and planning of the workshop.

It was decided that twelve people in any one group was the maximum for effective discussion; that three uninterrupted days would be needed to reach any useful conclusions; and that the principal interests to be represented were community service, health care, education, law, media, and policy analysis. Resources available were accommodation, air fares, meals, four project officers, four secretariat staff, four seminar rooms and a theatrette. It followed that there would be forty-eight participants, of whom four would be the DA:NA project officers. This left the difficult choice of forty-four people to represent six interest groups, eight States and Territories, four levels of action, fifteen principal ethnic groups, an unknown number of religions, a considerable range of drug problems and an age range from eighteen to sixty-five. In the event, these criteria of representation were met because the people chosen each wore three or four of these hats. The list of participants is included in the details of the workshop, attached as Appendix 1 of this chapter.

The DA:NA process is recorded in Figure 9. The workshop was to run from Sunday evening (time to learn the ropes, to settle in, to meet each other, to determine objectives and to check out personal agenda) to Wednesday lunchtime. Monday was allocated to exploring the options, Tuesday to agreeing on priorities and Wednesday to reaching agreement on the recommendations to go

A NATIONAL CAMPAIGN AGAINST DRUG ABUSE   179

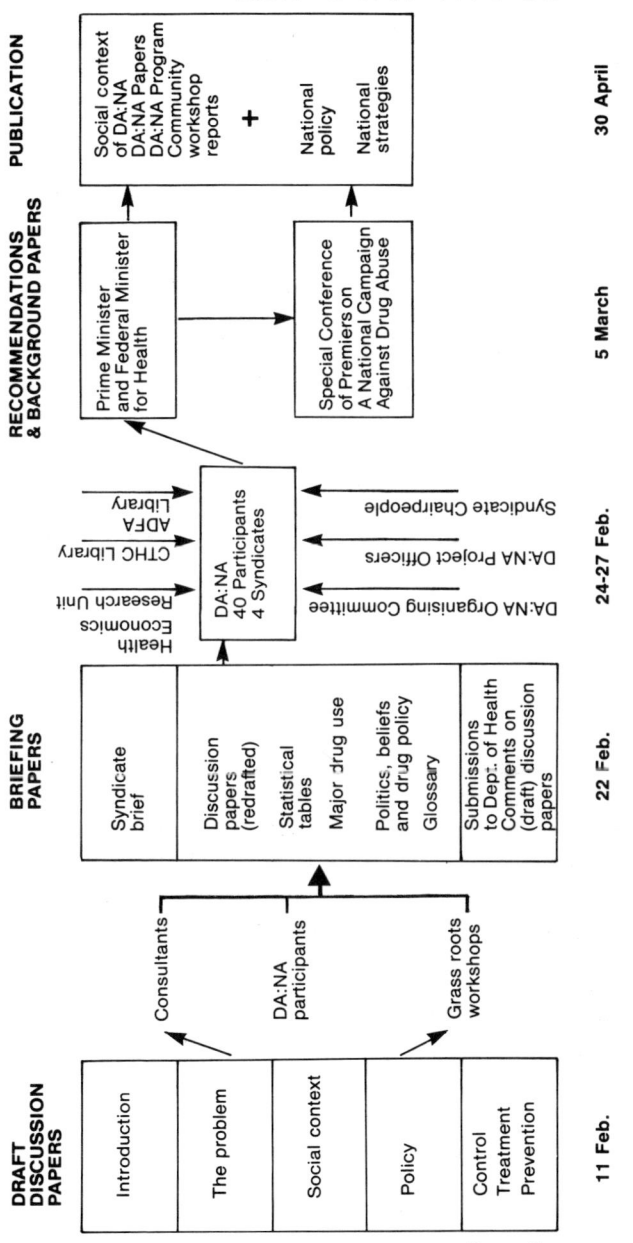

Figure 9   Framework for DA:NA

to the Drug Summit. The plan of the program is attached in Appendix 1; as one would expect, the workshop did not proceed as planned: group dynamics demand that such programs be flexible to adjust to needs as they arise, but the program as designed gives the goals and a guideline.

The rhythm of these three days was intended to be plenary, syndicate groups, plenary, syndicate groups, specialist advice, plenary, syndicate groups, and final plenary for ratification of recommendations. Not surprisingly, syndicates got out of phase with one another and the timetable was staggered and altered to their request. One result was that the final plenary did not provide time to consolidate all the recommendations, and this was done by an executive committee, appointed by workshop members.

A summary report with a short list of fifteen recommendations was conveyed to the Minister for Health, the Commonwealth Department of Health and the mass media on the day after the end of the workshop, Thursday 28 February. The full sixty-seven recommendations (attached in Appendix 1) followed later.

A full press conference was followed by interviews on radio and television, with a wide range of articles in national newspapers. This was important to keep the DA:NA recommendations in full view of public and politicians until the agenda for the Summit meeting was set, and during the Summit itself, so that the national community view was not forgotten.

The recommendations from the Summit also reflected those of the DA:NA workshop and of the previous major inquiries. One difference was that there was a three-year program with $60 million to put the recommendations into effect. A similarity was that the Summit again failed to deal with drug advertising, marijuana decriminalisation, or immigration control of drug runners.

Syndicate groups

The workshop was based on four syndicate working groups whose themes were to be the four sections of the action wheel described in Figure 1, namely, policy, social context, strategy, action. Briefing papers (redrafted as Chapters 2-8 of this book) provided a common content intended to forestall anyone in any one field from being 'the authority'. The papers were circulated to participants two weeks beforehand, to ensure that all participants had the chance to comment on the accuracy and comprehensiveness of the material. Every effort was made to use everyday language, to provide summary tables of up-to-date information and to design clear review charts on drug use.

The few formal presentations were the Commonwealth Minister for Health's welcome, the DA:NA Chairman's introduction, and brief contributions from four Members of the Federal Parliament. Excerpts of these last are included in Chapter 2, as examples of the social context in which the workshop was held.

Each of the four syndicate groups was led by a chairperson, serviced by a project officer and a secretary and one member of the Organising Committee.

Policy syndicate report
Agreement on specific strategies and action plans was much easier to achieve than agreement or even discussion on policy issues. Yet the problem with 'producing some sort of policy garment ... stitch by stitch' is that it leaves those people working on strategies and action plans in the dark as to what general approaches they should be taking. This is the complaint currently levelled at governments by on-the-ground agencies. It was certainly a difficulty with the Policy working group.

Social Context syndicate report
The Social Context syndicate group addressed the problems of fundamental social attitudes and of conditions which inhibit social change. It was agreed that if any strategic plan were to be effective, then the following social and structural impediments needed to be addressed: (a) trust/mistrust; (b) fear/ignorance; (c) dependence; (d) vested interests. Material from these discussions is presented in Chapter 2.

Strategy syndicate report
This group was engrossed in the identification of established, effective strategies. Of all the groups this was the most practical, one which came up with clear recommendations, and lent itself least to a descriptive report on group process. Task-centred from beginning to end, this group more than any other fulfilled its appointed task. Members divided into small groups to nominate strategies, and although debate on methadone as a maintenance

treatment, legalisation of cannabis, and control of prescribed drugs was strong, an effective compromise was reached in all cases, as the final recommendations show.

Action Plans syndicate report
This group was given the most practical brief. However, the members felt severely restricted by a feeling that they were not to discuss policy and several times voted to hold up discussion until the Policy syndicate could give them guidelines. Meanwhile, the groups proceeded to clarify and present extremely pertinent, focused and constructive recommendations on action, which were welcomed as a useful guide to their discussions by the other three syndicates.

Summary report of DA:NA

Policy recommendations from the workshop head the full list of recommendations attached as Appendix 1 to this chapter.

Areas of agreement were: the major drugs of abuse are alcohol and tobacco, heroin should not be legally provided, addicts should not be compelled to register, methadone is acceptable as one component of treatment, drug education is essential in schools and professions, family and community are the front line of prevention, a central database for co-ordination of information is urgently needed, use of media for public education should be encouraged, there should be drug rehabilitation within corrective services.

Four significant social trends emerged:

(a) while there are still the traditional polarised views on the use of drugs, there is now increasingly a common ground within the Australian community on appropriate action on the *abuse* of drugs

(b) there is growing acceptance that drug use includes many substances and that all people are potential users

(c) community forums are now dealing more readily with issues of demand for drugs but are not yet addressing issues of supply

(d) community opinion has moved away from stronger penalties for drug abuse towards rehabilitation and community education.

Evaluation of the DA:NA contribution to the Campaign

(a) *Empirical goals*: we have reviewed the process, proceedings and results of DA:NA. Recommendations were made on twelve of the sixteen empirical, observable items listed at the end of the workshop objectives, and all except the same four (enforced treatment, decriminalisation of marijuana, reducing criminal profits, and control of advertising) were also recommended from the Summit. The workshop contributed overall to the Summit by helping to set the agenda, by advising the Minister for Health on community opinion and by providing a framework which was reflected to a marked degree in the Summit recommendations (see Appendix 2 for comparisons).

(b) *Ethical goals*: these are expressed in the five statements issued by the Policy syndicate, and by the policy section of the sixty-seven recommendations. The chief goals can be identified as a concern for the balanced use of drugs, commitment to a strong community, education of the community on use and abuse, and protection of those at risk of abuse. In terms of Table 6, these goals are expressions of humanist and socialist policy positions. It is important to note, however, that business interests were thinly represented, and the laissez faire and conservative positions were not put forward.

(c) *Aesthetic standards*: this is the hidden aspect of most considerations in our society. Taste and feeling are not considered valid contributions to decision making, as they might be in either an eastern or a French community. There is no English equivalent of *ça va*. Strong rejections of some options were apparent and could well have been based on aesthetic judgments. Decisions on methadone seemed to be in this category, as did the decision on the control of media as a prevention strategy. Aesthetic distaste held by community workers and professionals for crime and corruption prevented the tackling of the principal issues connected with the supply of drugs.

(d) *Social rules*: the action and reaction within the workshop were, of course, within the social frameworks of the groups represented. Political realities were confrontations between professional roles and territories; and the meeting of social groups who normally have no chance to talk to each other. The 'norm' for policy advisers prevented them speaking in a public forum; youth and drug users were provided with their first forum (according to their own statement) in which they felt they had been heard. The presence of media representatives was of concern to some of the other professional groups. Prevention of abuse and reduction of demand were the principal strategy recommendations, as was to be expected from a community group selected for their reputation for social action.

Important changes in social rules recorded by the workshop are the four social trends listed in the Summary report. The first of these trends was illustrated by the workshop vote on the decriminalisation of marijuana: evenly split, with one-third for, against and undecided on the issue, yet all could vote for the expunging of criminal records after two years. Figure 9 reflects the degree of change since 1982 that this vote represents.

(e) *Individual range*: the moral positions on drug use held by workshop participants reflected the widely varied positions held in the community. People were evenly divided for and against the use of marijuana, on the basis of human rights for the former and the right to physical health for the latter. Methadone provides a similar split, the right to the treatment of choice against objection to social encouragement of controlled dependence. Strategies for education and community action were more strongly supported than those for increased treatment and control.

A personal commentary from one participant who had been there before is appended as a postscript to this book.

A grass roots community drug workshop

At the same time as the national community workshop was held in the national capital, more localised groups were meeting all over the country for the same purpose. There were policy workshops in most major States, whose recommendations varied, from those of New South Wales with an emphasis on legal constraints, increasing penalties and confiscating profits, to those of Western Australia which emphasised the need for education and community changes. Local community groups, who met more informally, were more likely to have drug abusers, families of abusers and treatment agencies at the same workshop.

One such community workshop was held in the same city, started on the same day, and used the same briefing papers as DA:NA. Local workers in the prevention and treatment of drug abuse felt shut out of the national initiative, and held a one-day seminar, open to all comers, to brief their local Member of Parliament to take their requests to DA:NA and, via the Minister for Health, to the Summit. Participants included professional workers from the local health authority and welfare services, members of voluntary organisations, users and self-defined abusers of legal and illegal drugs, parents of illegal drug users, members of local activist organisations, youth and women's shelters, workers in magistrates and higher courts, and representatives of local Members of Parliament and Councils. The breadth and the quantity of attendance reflected first, the interest held in the community for this issue, and second, the extent to which even a high-powered workshop in the same town at the same time is no replacement for a grass roots expression of local opinion.

The following is a summary of the recommendations of the Drug Abuse Seminar held in Canberra on Sunday, 24 February 1985. All recommendations were approved by a majority of those who attended, and on issues regarded as contentious a vote was taken. The results of such votes appear below the relevant recommendation.

Information and education
1. Institute a community information program (with special attention to teachers and parents) and a positive media campaign on what is involved in addiction, symptoms, avenues of assistance, and stressing that addicts can recover.
2. Training for drug counsellors and for all those professions that come into contact with addiction (lawyers, doctors, welfare workers, school counsellors, social workers), and for those already practising, provision of in-service training.
3. Education programs in schools to involve parents.
4. All health professionals should become informed about the adult children of addicts and about co-addiction.
5. Doctors should acknowledge the part they play in prescribed drug addiction.
6. Need for intervention in schools, as well as education.

7. All Community Health Centres should have drug and alcohol trained workers.
8. Research into and assessment of programs essential. Criteria for success essential.

Families
1. Need for recognition of the effects of addiction on families and family members: need assistance from qualified staff, encourage family participation and support in rehabilitation, acknowledge costs of addiction on families.

Law
1. Require a legislative change so that first offender drink drivers are sent to drug education programs.
2. Review legislation for alternatives to gaol for drug offenders, and institute counselling.
3. Lawyer/therapist relationship needs to be improved.
4. Assessment of addicts so that the legal system can deal adequately with addicts.
5. Sentencing options need to be widened enormously.
6. Supply free heroin to registered heroin addicts. (For 8; Against 5; Abstainers 5.)
7. Sentencing options for possession and personal use of presently illicit drugs should be reviewed and gaol or fine be excluded as an option. Institute counselling instead. (For 13; Against 1; Abstainers 5.)
8. Decriminalisation of cannabis and its derivatives, and reclassification. (For 12; Against 2; Abstainers 9.)

Local needs
1. Funding for staff for the Woden Valley Hospital detoxification centre.
2. Expansion of the methadone program.
3. Need for a non-medical detoxification centre.
4. Ensure that the ACT participates in the National Drug Education Program.
5. Finance for the expansion of Karralika in 1985-86 financial year.
6. Finance for the rural farm therapeutic community.
7. ACT to have its own Drug and Alcohol Authority on Northern Territory or Western Australian model.

8. ACT has drug problems just like the rest of Australia—recognition and funding for ACT would save New South Wales money.

Treatment and rehabilitation
1. Offer and fund a wide variety of rehabilitation options, recognising that drug abuse has many causes and manifestations, and recovery approaches also need to provide variety.
2. Urgent need for a first point of contact for those with drug problems, especially outside business hours.
3. Management of addiction should be considered seriously.
4. Need for alternatives to medical treatment.
5. More relevant counselling for those on methadone maintenance and funding of counsellors, some of whom to be ex-addicts.
6. Need for minor tranquilliser clinics to be established in all Community Health Centres.
7. Recognition that women require special treatment, and that childcare facilities be provided.
8. Halfway houses for recovering alcoholics and other drug users.
9. Treatment for nicotine addiction.
10. Basis for ongoing funding of treatment and rehabilitation centres to be evaluation of programs.

These recommendations are noteworthy for their direct address to action, in contrast to those of the national workshop, which presented solely policy and strategy options. The two sets together provide a comprehensive package. Both called for recognition of concern about the present use of legal drugs, community support, education of children, parents and professionals, and more rehabilitation services. The two are in disagreement on only the following issues: tougher legislation for first offenders, with alternatives to gaol; registration and assessment of addicts; heroin supplied to addicts; responsibilities of health professionals.

A State community drug workshop

State and local community workshops, by definition, reflect the immediate concerns of their area or locality. One State workshop, that of New South Wales, attended by two hundred people ranging from academics to prostitutes and drug addicts, was given a more formal agenda than the previous two workshops discussed. Formal papers were followed by comment from an invited panel. Themes chosen were not dissimilar from those in Part 2 of this book, namely The Problem in Context, Treatment and Rehabilitation, Law Enforcement, Prevention and Education, and Research and Policy Options.

Not surprisingly, each section contained both speakers who urged considerable increases in resources for their own area and critics of the present level of achievement in the same area. *Connexions,* the newsletter of drug and alcohol services in New South Wales, provides a practical review of the contributions and the subsequent discussion; the issue of March-April 1985 provides a valuable snapshot of the agreement and disagreement of professionals in each of the theme areas. It seems appropriate to leave the summing up in the hands of the State Premier, Neville Wran.

> A number of contributors put forward new strategies or ideas that had particular value. These included establishing a National Institute for Drug and Alcohol Studies; setting up 24-hour drug and alcohol detoxification services for women, children and youth; increasing peer support programmes within schools; improving existing drug education programmes for parents, teachers and professionals; and providing more funds for Australian research so as not to rely on overseas findings which may not be relevant. Other ideas contained implications for State policies and these will be considered by the Government in the light of strategies and actions determined at the Summit.
>
> Some submissions expressed support for or opposition to issues such as controls on the use of cannabis, use of methadone as a treatment option, availability of methadone programmes, advertising of alcohol, accreditation of non-government agencies, responsibilities of pharmaceutical companies about the effects of prescription drugs, controls on the prescription of barbiturates by doctors, stricter penalties for drug 'pushers' and provision of heroin to registered users.
>
> There were also submissions which sought more funding for an expansion of existing services. These related mainly to treatment and rehabilitation services, while others mentioned education and research needs. All these proposals will be evaluated further, following the Premiers' Conference.

Submissions from the general public

The Prime Minister and the Federal Minister for Health advertised for people to submit their ideas, so that the National Campaign could reflect community concerns.

The following summary is the work of Jean Nolan and others from the Commonwealth Department of Health.

> 507 submissions were received.
>
> Most of the submissions were concerned with the illegal use of drugs. However, 14 per cent mentioned that they considered the national strategy or campaign should include alcohol and/or tobacco. Of these, a number recommended a variety of measures in relation to alcohol and tobacco and emphasised the problems associated with the use of these drugs. One organisation indicated that alcohol should not be included in the campaign as it was a different drug from the 'illicit' drugs.
>
> The majority of submissions were from people with 'extreme' views, with a direct personal involvement, or who were working in associated areas, e.g. treatment, rehabilitation, education, etc. However, there were a large number of submissions from individuals in the community who felt they should express their views and, overall, most respondents appeared to have a genuine desire to contribute to the National Campaign.
>
> 110 submissions were received from government or non-government organisations, 2 from business firms offering assistance and 395 from individuals. Following their initial submissions, 14 respondents each sent in further submissions.
>
> Among the individuals, 39 volunteered that they belonged to the medical profession, paramedical professions or alternative medicine; 31 indicated they were addicts or ex-addicts, while 42 were parents, other relatives or friends of addicts. 13 indicated that they belonged to the teaching profession, 6 to law enforcement groups and 3 were ministers of religion. Apart from organisations, 18 submissions were from individuals working in drug prevention, treatment or rehabilitation areas.

Media coverage of national drug issues

In the Australian press between November 1984 and June 1985, there was hardly a day in any newspaper in which drug issues were not raised. Television was more uneven, but the subject was certainly not ignored. National commentators and current affairs programs kept the pot boiling. That last is a rather weak pun;

cannabis was a favourite for headlines, with heroin seizures second, and allusions to big crime about third. One newspaper ran a regular column called 'The drug debate', and national magazines rarely omitted an article on the Drug Campaign.

Responses to the announcement of the Campaign varied from 'about time' to 'a political whitewash'. Press comments on the recommendations were disappointment and some criticism that the cannabis issue was unresolved and surprise that control and registration of addicts had not been further considered (although community groups had spoken strongly against these). The expansion of the methadone maintenance program was in general treated as simple justice, without much recognition of the issues involved. But the overwhelming point taken from the Campaign by the Australian press was the recognition that alcohol and nicotine were real causes for concern. A difficult issue for both media and politicians because of the excise and advertising revenue involved, alcohol and nicotine nevertheless claimed their share of the headlines.

Table 25

Ranking of thematic content by press and television, Sydney area 1984

Rank	Press	Television	Total
1	Political	Political	Political
2	Res/Opinion	Crime Syndicate	Res/Opinion
3	Health	Res/Opinion	Crime Syndicate
4	Industry	Drug Busts	Health
5	Prev/Education	Drug Seizures	Industry
6	Crime Syndicate	Health	Drug Busts
7	Drug Busts	Industry	Prevention/Education
8	Advertising	Prev/Education	Advertising
9	Sports	Agencies	Drug Seizures
10	Agencies	Advertising	Agencies
11	History	Sport and History	Sports
12	Seizures	Drug/Drive	History
13	Drug/Drive		Drug/Drive

Source: Reprinted by permission of CEIDA, from *Connexions* 5(2) March-April 1985, p.8

An analysis of the Sydney media treatment of drug issues has been issued by the Centre for Education and Information on Drugs and Alcohol (CEIDA), and builds on a previous report of 1982 media by Philip Bell. Bell had identified a focus on drug-crime links, with a tendency to report in hero-villain style. Current (1985) reporting emphasises the political implications and health and industrial consequences of drug abuse. While television continues to concentrate on the cannabis-crime bust theme, newspaper articles on drug themes have doubled in the last two years, with emphasis on comment and drugs as a social issue. The ranking of drug-related issues and storyline themes can be seen in Tables 25 and 26. In terms of the social issues involved, it could be fairly said that the media reflected a move from 'it's us and them, and drug abusers are them' to consideration of general influences on politics and health of the country, a major shift which it would be difficult to interpret as either leader or follower of political and/or public opinion. It seems reasonable to conclude that all three reached the same point at the same time.

Table 26

Major drug stories of 1984 in Sydney media

Drug stories were more prevalent in the latter half of 1984 (1288 items between January and June; 1882 items between July and December). Major stories for the year were:

Mackay inquest	March
Leukemia drug story	June
Trimbole/Mackay	October
Corruption, NSW police	October
Alcohol advertising	October
Trimbole	November
Costigan Reports	November
Operation Noah	November
Operation Triangle	December (Marijuana raids)
Random breath testing	December
Operation Noah	December
Kings Cross heroin	December

Source: Reprinted by permission of CEIDA, from *Connexions* 5(2) March-April 1985, p.8

The quintessence of the National Campaign

Views on drug use and abuse from almost every category of Australian citizen (it is hard to think of any excluded), goals of our decision makers from Prime Minister and judges to union officials, estimates of abuse from all the Australian material available, and the aspects of drug use which interest the Australian public have all been gathered in relation to the National Campaign Against Drug Abuse (NCADA). These now supply a baseline, a 'before' measure for a before and after evaluation of the Campaign.

Physical background

There seems no doubt that, among the various drugs of abuse, the single greatest cause of social disruption and unhappiness is the over-consumption of alcohol; while the greatest cause of ill health and death is nicotine. There seems no doubt that the overuse of prescription tranquillisers and barbiturates is an iceberg of which we see only the tip, but a tip which seems to be diminishing. There seems no doubt that our children have access to all the adult drugs, as young as they wish to try them, and that use is begun between 9 and 11 years of age.

There seems no doubt that our society supports a massive black economy in, not only the newsworthy cannabis, but prescription drugs and synthetic moodchangers. Heroin, which seems to act as the totem for all illicit drugs, is used by comparatively few (about 3 per cent?), but these few are likely to be already at risk from other drug use, and to extend the criminal element in society to a point where the law enforcement systems are called into question. The general use of cocaine in the drug scene has only just reached Australia; its progress is too early to chart. Over-prescription of drugs for the aged is suspected, but not regarded as proven. Self-dosing by women with analgesics in epidemic proportions is proven, and is just showing a decline.

Ethical goals

The bases on which policy can be formulated are the statements of principle assembled from those made during the lead-up to the Summit, by politicians and citizens alike.

The Australian community and the family, as institutions which cannot be allowed to be threatened, emerged very strongly as statements of principle. The rights of different groups, and of each individual, in pursuit of control, treatment, education or community development, were to be ensured. The often suggested labels of 'the learning society' or 'the information society' for our era are reflected in the emphasis on education as a desirable strategy, and in the calls for a strong research capacity. Control and treatment are seen as necessary, but not sufficient; the opportunity for the individual to return as a 'normal' individual to a 'normal' life is a strong requirement placed on those services.

In reviewing these value positions, we have already remarked that they reflect socialist and liberal humanist value positions. Yet competition and laissez faire are also strong values in our society, as are Christian values which might direct us towards change to a better society. The former positions may well be reflected in the creation of the drug-based fortunes—everyone is entitled to do the best they can for themselves.

The ethical requirement for the professions to treat the drug-addicted with dignity was put forward by the grass roots workshop, and the moral responsibility to forcibly treat and to punish was put forward in the individual submissions. Surprisingly, in what has been called a child-centred society, and with the evidence of early child use of drugs, there were no strong emphases given to protection of children, although there were many recommendations for education as the major preventive strategy.

Aesthetic standards

The strong influences *for* the taking of drugs were rarely, if ever, mentioned. The acceptance of alcohol, nicotine, marijuana (among about 10 per cent of the population) and caffeine as inducing desirable physical and aesthetic responses was either taken for granted or ignored. The lack of mention of these community standards can give a somewhat unrealistic air to the drug debate. Nevertheless, it is possible to discern some aesthetic standards in the control measures as well. The clean, tidy nature of treatment as an option is aesthetically preferable to the bleakness of a prison or the scruffiness of a community agency. These tastes, apparent in many of the submissions, contrast with the more intellectualised recommendations which point out the virtues of co-ordinated community action and peer support.

The inconsistencies in response to the risks of different drugs must surely have some roots in the aesthetic senses. How else to explain the real revulsion against marijuana, a drug whose physical effects are no worse than nicotine, to say the least, and whose emotional effect is no stronger than that of alcohol? Or the acceptance of daily doses of caffeine above the medical stimulant dose (which is only about five cups of tea or coffee), but the taboo on admitting that other medical doses, of tranquillisers or amphetamines, are taken for pleasure?

Aesthetic standards in drug taking are rarely mentioned or taken into account, and yet provide one of the strongest pressures to abuse, or to avoid, chemical changes of consciousness. Aesthetic standards therefore provide a potentially strong agent in the prevention of abuse.

Social rules

In the summary of DA:NA, we noted four changes in social rules: namely, the shift to accepting alcohol as a drug of abuse, as well as an Australian social totem; the acceptance that all Australians are potentially drug users, and so open to the risk of drug abuse; the change from an emphasis on control to an emphasis on education as a preferred preventive strategy; and finally, agreement on drugs as a threat to Australian society. These are all highly significant in terms of importance to the social framework, significant enough to confirm that we live in an era of social change, and that Mead's prefigurative society has been brought to pass. For the older members of society these changes could well be impossible to accept; for the young they are not changes but the stuff of which their world is made.

Another method of determining social rules is to look at the CEIDA analysis of the headline stories; presumably these main stories indicate a break in the normal pattern of social activities, a 'man bites dog' phenomenon.

In this light, reviewing Table 26, we can discern an interaction between totem and taboo. Taboo is the murder of a responsible citizen (Mackay); totem is the use of drugs to halt dread diseases (leukemia); taboo is the idea of law enforcement officers being criminal; taboo is the idea of the great marketing miracle, advertising, being used to sell harmful substances; and a totem is a Royal Commission whose findings create reality out of rumour. The documentation of the breaking of a totem or a taboo, or the creation of new totems or fresh taboos, is one way of evaluating the course of the National Campaign.

Individual perspectives
We have seen the range of individual moral positions, and aesthetic standards, and the mixture of social rules in the area of drug use and abuse. Measures of the present positions are available, as are the measures of rates and effects of use and abuse. Where do we go from here is now the question; or rather, given that the ethical goals have been clearly stated, the need to balance use and abuse recognised, and the social rules involved identified, the question should be—can we get there from here?

Appendix 1:
DA:NA Workshop

(A) Recommendations,
(B) Participants,
(C) Workshop design

(A) DA:NA RECOMMENDATIONS
General Policy

Objective
1. The objective of a national policy on drug use should be to minimise the harmful consequences of the use of drugs to individuals, their families, and the community as a whole including the needs of special groups. Therefore a national, comprehensive approach will be required.

General principles
2. All drugs which may lead to dependence or be abused should be included in a national policy on drugs. In particular, the policy should acknowledge that alcohol and tobacco are the major drugs of use and abuse in Australia and they should be a major focus of attention in the forthcoming national action.

3. In general the overall level of use of drugs of dependence in the community is related to the level of harm associated with the use of these drugs, therefore a national strategy should aim to reduce the overall level of use of all such drugs.

4. Individuals differ widely in their drug use patterns, their reactions to these and their need for support; there is a multiplicity of drugs being abused in the community. This diversity should be recognised in a national policy on drug abuse.

5. Where drug programs are developed to suit the needs of a distinct group of people, whether they be 'disadvantaged' or a naturally occurring client group, these people should be involved in the program design, implementation and evaluation.

6. Primary prevention is paramount and should receive a high priority in formulation of policy and in funding.

7. Governments should acknowledge through financial and other support the value of non-government programs.

8. Reliable information concerning drug use and abuse, including information relevant to the special needs of particular groups and communities, should be readily available.

9. Research, evaluation and the development of national databases must be an essential part of a national drug policy, both with respect to the development and management of programs and the administration of drug controls.

10. There should be a policy to increase the level of awareness within the Australian community of the potential benefits of some use of some drugs, and the potential for harm of all drugs..

11. A national policy will need to recognise the cultural, social, family and behavioural predispositions to all drug use.

12. The use of drugs should be examined and policies developed within a perception of the historical context of drug use.

Strategies for prevention, control and treatment

(i) Community

13. Community development strategies should be developed and implemented, in order to improve and/or change the social environment which promotes and reinforces drug-taking behaviour.

14. Traditional and urban Aboriginal communities and family groups have special needs. The burden of drug misuse is high and while rehabilitation services receive some financial support, there are few preventive services. As a general strategy, the people concerned must be involved in all stages of program design, implementation and evaluation. Preventive services must be increased and emphasis placed on community-based schemes (also note Recommendation 5).

15. Special priority should be given to funding programs of a preventive nature which provide alternatives to drug use.

16. Government should co-operate with other major organisations to promote effective and evaluated programs which are not drug-specific but which promote self-esteem and skills in self-sufficiency.
17. Tax incentives should be offered to industries providing funds to approved drug abuse programs.

Families

18. Since families have an important role in the prevention, early detection and treatment of drug abuse, they should be enabled to fulfil this role by:

    the provision of easily available and relevant information through health services, educational institutions and other appropriate outlets

    access to workers trained to provide family therapy in relation to drugs

    recognition of the contribution that can be made by self-help groups of family members to the prevention of emotional and physical trauma and to public education on drugs

    encouragement of formation of self-help groups in local areas.

(ii) Education

19. Education programs about drugs and their social setting should permeate the whole educational process, including the education of professional people.
20. Education, at all levels, should include programs which prepare people to make more informed decisions about lifestyle (e.g. problem solving, decision making) and should be part of the standard curriculum.
21. Drug education in schools should be strengthened.

    (a) This education process needs to be within the curriculum, preferably within health and human relations courses, and be linked with community activities and local services.

    (b) This education program should be extended to a broad range of community groups and not limited to special target groups.

    (c) Educative interventions should aim to provide participants with the opportunity and skills to create an environment of appropriate drug use.

22. Information and educative resources need to be provided as important support services within the community. This could be integrated into general health promotion services.

23. Persons or authorities responsible for drug education programs should consult with Education Departments to design learning kits and units of work across the broad range of drug issues.

24. The student unit of drug education should commence in preparatory class and continue through primary and secondary school.

25. Health and Education Departments should have a commitment to:

    teacher training in substance abuse issues
    production of teaching guides
    development of strategies to convince school administrators about the importance of substance abuse education
    the involvement of parents, where appropriate
    in-service training.

26. Special professional training at all levels, including medical schools, is required. In particular:

    (a) Professional (postgraduate and continuing) education, related to drugs, including primary prevention, needs to be available and at the highest possible standard for all health, welfare and police and correctional service personnel.

    (b) The role of all health and welfare professionals in the process of early identification and intervention needs to be defined and appropriate training given to meet these needs.

    (c) Staff involved in the management of all types of drug problems should be enabled to have regular and relevant staff development and professional updating through appropriate in-service training, and postgraduate training through special courses should be provided in tertiary institutions with specially dedicated funds.

27. Evaluation of all education strategies should be undertaken, to ensure effectiveness in achieving stated goals.

(iii) Law Enforcement

28. Such profits and assets of individuals and corporations as are accumulated through illicit drug trading should be confiscated legally, and should be applied in such proportion as is deemed appropriate by government for use in drug management programs.

29. We recommend, for drug users, the option of diversion from the legal system to treatment when appropriate facilities are available and acceptable to the individual. Where adequate facilities do not exist they should be made available.

30. We recommend the establishment of an assessment process for those before the courts on drug-related charges through a team that will screen and assess individuals enabling recommendations to be made to the court that will assist the court in sentencing, and the individual in gaining appropriate treatment.

31. Licensing restrictions are an important form of control in alcohol sales and need close evaluation and should be regularly reviewed and related to community needs and health considerations.

32. The illicit drug trade can generate corruption in every area of society. Recognising that this problem must be tackled at all levels, one obvious need is to ensure that direct law enforcement authorities each have fully empowered, adequately staffed internal investigatory bodies, with proper pursuit of convictions through the courts.

33. Special prescription forms for doctors to supply dangerous drugs (colour coded, serial numbered) should be introduced nationally.

34. Research into the relationships between drug abuse and crime must be supported and developed through the appropriate national and State research agencies.

35. Amongst the means available to influence the consumption of alcohol and tobacco, the following are recommended for implementation:

    (a) The introduction of differential taxation reflecting the alcohol content of beverages and the tar content of cigarettes.

    (b) An increase in real terms of the price of alcoholic beverages and tobacco and the price of alcoholic beverages and tobacco to be regularly reviewed in line with increases in the CPI so that their price, relative to disposable income, remains constant.

    (c) The introduction of random breath testing in all States and Territories and the standardisation of the permissible blood alcohol level at 0.05.

    (d) The review and revision of all crimes and penalties relating to alcohol and tobacco sale and use, with a view to ascertaining and improving their efficacy in reducing the harm associated with these drugs.

    (e) Whilst the advertising of alcohol and tobacco remains, interpretation of the present voluntary codes is to be vested in bodies on which health and other consumer interests are adequately represented.

(iv) Media and Information

36. Media campaigns play an important part in public health. They must be directed at well-identified target groups and have clear objectives. This Workshop supports the use of media campaigns where the above criteria are met and where local needs are adequately taken into account through consultation, research and evaluation.

37. No mass media program on drugs, either at a Commonwealth or State level, should be undertaken without some evidence of potential success, and in the case of Commonwealth campaigns consultation with all State Health Departments.

38. Wherever appropriate, a mass media program should have back-up support programs at a local level, built-in evaluation, adequate funding.

39. Liaison with the media should be pursued with a view to establishing guidelines for reporting substance-related matters.

40. Closer collaboration between the communication media, education, and law enforcement should be encouraged.

41. All forms of advertising of tobacco should be banned, and a statutory code should be developed (replacing the present voluntary code) governing the advertising of alcohol. The interpretation of this should be vested in a body on which health, road safety and other consumer groups are adequately represented.

42. There should be an investigation into the design of legislation which requires compensatory advertising paid for by drug and alcohol advertisers or, alternatively, by government.

43. Sponsorship of sporting events based on the promotion of alcohol and tobacco should be phased out.

44. Properly planned and co-ordinated public education programs (via media and health promotion) should be implemented:

    to establish that the drug problem is everyone's problem

    to demystify community beliefs and attitudes

    to provide information and resources

    to assist communities to set agenda

    to foster an awareness of cultural differences

    to foster recognition that harm from legal drugs is greater than from illegal

    to create an understanding that drug problems are rarely caused solely by drug usage to raise community awareness that there is no 'quick fix'

to increase public awareness of drug treatment programs which promote greater public acceptance of drug users and which counter their alienation from the community.

(v) Research and Resources

45. A national centre or institute of drug studies should be established with the following functions:
    (a) to develop, evaluate and utilise data systems on drugs
    (b) to evaluate social policy
    (c) to initiate basic and applied research into drugs and the treatment of dependence
    (d) to develop model cross-disciplinary education, training and treatment programs
    (e) to promote exchange of ideas between professions and communities in Australia
    (f) to provide a model of support and co-ordination of community drug programs developed by communities
    (g) to provide a consultancy service—e.g. promote a public climate of co-operation between governments, media and the community.

46. The national centre should include the full range of relevant disciplines and the directorship should be drawn from any appropriate discipline. The centre should be adequately funded to enable it to achieve world standing.

47. No special State or national registers of drug users should be established; however, usual requirements for registration of patients in treatment programs, and registration required in the dispensing of certain drugs, are acceptable.

48. To provide essential information the following studies are required:
    (a) a national longitudinal study of drug use
    (b) drug use surveys on a regular basis, across all age groups and across all drugs
    (c) systematic audits on particular social indicators related to drug use.

49. A national institute should record all results of evaluation of treatment, educational and preventive programs.

50. An Australian modification of the client-oriented data acquisition process (CODAP) should be developed.

(vi) Treatment and Rehabilitation
51. Programs for drug users should be accredited and the guidelines for accreditation should include levels of care such as:
    (a) A person considered for inclusion in any treatment program should have access to full information and counselling about the nature of the program.
    (b) Where any person requires admission into a treatment program she/he has a right to well-maintained clinics and rehabilitation services, and access twenty-four hours a day to a counselling service and crisis intervention.
    (c) A wide range of interventions aimed at assisting individuals manifesting harmful drug behaviours should be provided.
    (d) Community programs should be part of the community, staffed by community members and legitimised by involvement of local community leaders.
52. Evaluation measures and procedures should be mandatory for all treatment programs.
53. Prescribed addictive and/or mind-altering drugs should be accompanied by appropriate and accurate information on the consequences of their use.
54. Adequate funding should be provided in the areas of treatment and rehabilitation, including non-government programs.
55. Rehabilitation programs for those in custody for offences involving drug dependence should be actively promoted and supported in corrective services throughout Australia.
56. Rehabilitation programs must be an integral element of the corrective institution and be integrated into the institutional philosophy and policy.
57. Every prisoner convicted of a drug-related offence should be assessed and evaluated psychologically and educationally by use of appropriate test and clinical interviews administered by qualified professionals, and this should become an integral part of normal prison operations prior to allocation to an appropriate rehabilitation program.
58. In the management of heroin addiction, legal provision of heroin should not be part of the national drug policy.

59. Some participants expressed reservations about the use of methadone as a treatment at any time. Others expressed reservations about expansion in the use of methadone as a panacea for heroin problems. However, all agreed that:

> In the management of heroin addiction, methadone programs (both withdrawal and maintenance) should be supported as one of a variety of methods (such as therapeutic communities, ongoing counselling and outpatients drug-free programs) available to those who are opiate dependents.

60. Existing national guidelines for the use of methadone should be revised in the light of recommendations 59, 61 and 62.

61. National funding of methadone maintenance programs should be conditional on the programs' operating within agreed minimum standard requirements.

62. Adequate research should be undertaken to determine what priority should be given to funding methadone programs, if it is determined additional national support should be given.

63. A national education campaign, taking into account the needs of special groups, should be run to inform addicts and the public of the nature and aim of any proposed methadone program and the possible success rate.

64. Opinion amongst participants was almost equally divided between liberal and conservative points of view in relation to cannabis. Nevertheless, the following recommendation was accepted unanimously:

> The criminal records of those convicted of possession for personal use should be destroyed at the end of two years, on the application of the person convicted, except in stipulated circumstances; access to such records should be restricted to members of law enforcement agencies, and to authorities having lawful access to police records for criminological research.

65. Further research/monitoring of the use of cannabis is needed in order to evaluate long-term effects.

66. Research is needed on the levels of impairment of performance under the influence of cannabis and development is needed of simple equipment for an accurate test for driving under the influence of cannabis.

67. Community education campaigns are needed which provide accurate information concerning the use and abuse of cannabis.

(B) DA:NA PARTICIPANTS

ANDREWS, Miss Rhyan
Student Initiatives in Community Health
Sydney

BAILEY, Ms Leila
Counselling Service
Australian National University
Canberra

BALDWIN, Mr Richard
Drug and Alcohol Policy Analyst
Department of Health
Sydney

BURNS, Dr F. Harding
Alcohol and Drug Foundation, Australia
Sydney

CHESHER, Dr G.B.
Psychopharmacology Research Unit
Sydney

DEVESON, Ms Anne
Dulwich, Adelaide

DUNN, Dr Sydney
Werribee, Victoria

FARMER, Mr Richard
Journalist and wine merchant
Canberra

FOSTER, Dr Alan
Alcohol and Drug Foundation, Australia
Hobart

GARNER, Mr Gerry
Family Living
Adelaide

HACKETT, Dr Earle
Adelaide

HAWKS, Professor David
Western Australian Drug and Alcohol Authority
Perth

HERMES, Mr C.
Magistrate, ACT

HOLLINGSWORTH, Mr Bill
Alcohol and Drug Foundation, Australia
Cairns

JANS, Mrs Jean
Community Approach to Drug Abuse Prevention
Canberra

KALUCY, Professor Ross
Flinders University
Adelaide

KEATING, Mr John
WANAD
The Holyoake Institute
Perth

KERR, Professor C.B.
Department of Preventive and Social Medicine
Institute of Health
Sydney

MANNING, Mr R.W.
Pharmacist, Canberra

MOON, Dr John
Alcohol and Drug Foundation, Victoria
Melbourne

MORISON, Ms Sarah
Workers with Youth Network
Canberra

MYKOLAJENKO, Mr Tony
Private psychologist
Sydney

NOFFS, Reverend Ted
Wayside Chapel
Sydney

NOLAN, Mr D.
Confederation of Australian
    Industry
Canberra

PANNELL, Mr B.W.
Director Intelligence
Australian Customs Service
Canberra

PARFITT, Dr R.T.
Principal
Canberra College of Advanced
    Education
Canberra

POWELL, Dr K
Director
Alcohol and Drug Service
Drug Dependence Unit
Woden Valley Hospital
Canberra

REDPATH, Mr Bill
International Youth Year
    Secretariat
Canberra

SANTAMARIA, Dr J.N.
Director
Autumn School of Studies
    on Alcohol and Drugs
St Vincent's Hospital
Melbourne

SARGEANT, Mrs Delys
Social Biology Resources Centre
Melbourne

SCUTT, Dr Jocelynne A.
Law Reform Commission of
    Victoria
Melbourne

STEPHENS, Ms Lynda
Health Promotion Unit
Victorian Health Commission
Melbourne

STEUR, Ms Mel
Senior Research Officer
Biala
Brisbane

STEWART, The Hon. Mr
    Justice D.G.
National Crime Authority
Sydney

STONE, Mr Ken
ACTU Representative
Victorian Trades Hall Council
Melbourne

SUMMERS, Dr Anne
First Assistant Secretary
Office of the Status of Women
Canberra

SUTTON, Dr Jeff
Director
Bureau of Crime Statistics
    and Research
Sydney

TRINCA, Mr Gordon
Road Trauma Committee
College of Surgeons
Melbourne

VULCAN, Dr Peter
Road Safety and Traffic
  Management Bureau
Melbourne

WARDLAW, Mr Grant
Australian Institute of
  Criminology
Canberra

WHEELWRIGHT, Assoc.
  Prof. E.L.
Economics, University of Sydney
Sydney

WHITE, Ms Kate
Banyan House
Darwin

WORTHY, Detective
  Superint. L.
Australian Federal Police
Canberra

Politicians

BAUME, Senator The Hon.
  Peter E.
Commonwealth Parliament
  Office
Sydney

BLEWETT, The Hon. Neal
Commonwealth Minister for
  Health
Parliament House
Barton, ACT

CROWLEY, Senator Rosemary
Adelaide

KELLY, Mrs Roslyn J.
Bonner House
Phillip, ACT

(C) DA:NA WORKSHOP DESIGN

Day 1, Sunday, 24 February	Information, Welcome. Minister for Health and DA:NA Chairman
Day 2, Monday, 25 February	Identifying the options for a National Drug Campaign
Day 3, Tuesday, 26 February	Drafting conclusions and recommendations
Day 4, Wednesday, 27 February	Ratifying recommendations to Special Conference of Premiers

Day 1: Sunday 1, 24 February: Welcome to DA:NA

4.00 pm Registration for interstate guests, University House, ANU.
5.30 pm Organising Committee's welcome to participants.
6.45 pm Dinner (seated in syndicate groups—the working groups for the workshop).
8.00 pm Informal welcome—Federal Minister for Health, the Honourable Neal Blewett and DA:NA Chairman, Professor Ian Webster.
8.30 pm Participants' expectations of workshop.
9.00 pm Close

Day 2: Monday, 25 February: Identifying options for a National Drug Strategy

8.30 am DA:NA Chairman—Review of objectives and timetable for workshop.
9.00 am Official opening—Minister for Health, the Honourable Neal Blewett.
9.30 am *Syndicate Working Group 1*
    Tasks: Clarify objectives of workshop
            Identify working schedule
             Establish areas of agreement, disagreement
             Identify new ideas, new solutions
10.30 am Morning Tea
11.00 am *Syndicate Working Group 2*
    Tasks: Relate objectives to syndicate theme
            Identify these problem areas and options
1.00 pm Lunch
2.00 pm Plenary session: Reporting panel—five chairpeople
2.30 pm Personal: Participants write personal briefing notes.
2.45 pm *Syndicate Working Group 3*
    Tasks: Rework syndicate theme options in light of plenary
            Identify unsolved issues and areas of insufficient information and/or disagreement
3.30 pm Afternoon Tea
4.00 pm *Syndicate Working Group 4*
    Tasks: Establish outline of issues to be dealt with by Special Conference of Premiers
            Establish list of viable options for solutions
            Identify areas for further information
6.00 pm Dinner
7.00 pm Material for proposed media campaign (theatrette)

7.30 pm *Syndicate Working Group 5*
          Tasks: Draft outline of recommendations on syndicate theme
8.45 pm Buses leave Capital Territory Health Commission

Day 3: Tuesday, 26 February: Conclusions and Recommendations
8.30 am Members of Parliament
9.30 am Panel of requested specialists (plenary and/or syndicate)
10.30 am Morning Tea
11.00 am Special interest groups: issues outstanding
12.00 pm *Syndicate Working Group 6*
          Tasks: Definition of principles
                 Proposals for recommendations
1.00 pm Lunch
2.00 pm *Syndicate Working Group 7*
          Tasks: Drafting of conclusions and recommendations
                 Time for personal review
3.15 pm Afternoon Tea
3.45 pm Plenary: Syndicate chairpeople present recommendations (distributed in typed form)
6.00 pm Reception
8.30 pm Buses leave CTHC

Day 4: Wednesday, 27 February: Ratifying Recommendations
9.00 am *Syndicate Working Group 8*
          Tasks: Completed recommendations for Special Conference of Premiers
10.00 am Plenary: Recommendations proposed
10.30 am Morning Tea
11.00 am Special purpose groups
11.30 am Plenary: Recommendations ratified
12.30 pm Press conference for Minister for Health and DA:NA Chairman
12.30 pm Lunch

Appendix 2:

Official Release from the Special Premiers' Conference on Drugs, Canberra, 2 April 1985

The Commonwealth, State and Territory Heads of Government met in Canberra in a special Premiers' Conference and pledged their governments to do everything possible to combat the growing problems of drug abuse and addiction in Australia. They agreed to mount a National Campaign Against Drug Abuse in which all governments will co-operate and which will also seek the full involvement and support of the community as a whole.

The Campaign will place a major emphasis on reducing the demand for drugs through education, treatment and rehabilitation programs, particularly for young people and particularly relating to hard drugs.

The Conference noted that the cost to the Australian community of drug abuse is high whether measured in terms of death and illness, wasted human potential, violent and property crime, loss of production or social misery. It was recognised that drug abuse is a complex problem and that there are no simple or quick solutions. The Conference agreed that a sustained effort would be required over a period of years.

The Conference emphasised that governments have a special responsibility to address problems associated with those drugs the use of which is illegal in our society. It was agreed that the Campaign will focus particularly on illegal drugs. At the same time it was recognised that there are also widespread health and social problems arising from the abuse of licit drugs and that the Campaign will need to encompass these as well.

The Conference agreed that it was essential that government efforts to combat drug trafficking and to prevent supplies of hard drugs coming into the country be intensified. Particular attention will be paid to those who control, direct and finance such activities.

The Conference recognised, however, that the drug problem will not be effectively tackled unless there is success in reducing the demand for drugs.

Every effort will be made to convince young people of the dangers of involvement with drugs. Greater assistance and support will be provided for parents, educators, community groups and others who work with and counsel young people. It was also agreed that both the quality and the quantity of treatment and rehabilitation programs for those already suffering from drug addiction should be improved.

Special attention will be given to the needs of particular sectors of the community. The so called hard drugs pose a threat to young people generally: but for other groups, such as Aborigines, abuse of licit drugs, or substances, may be more significant problems.

The Conference acknowledged that women's pattern of drug use differs from men's and presents problems which may require different approaches. There are particular problems which need to be addressed in the case of heroin-addicted women who may be forced into prostitution or, in the case of pregnant addicts, whose lives and those of their babies may be endangered. The Conference also noted the greater reliance of women on minor tranquillisers and agreed that measures were needed to dissuade doctors and patients from resorting to these drugs of addiction.

The Commonwealth Government will contribute to the Campaign by the funding of national projects and by making additional funds available to the States. The States and the Northern Territory will continue to expand existing programs, provide matching funds and administer a major part of Commonwealth funding.

The Commonwealth Government has committed itself to a long-term program of assistance. For the next three years it has agreed to provide up to an additional $20 million a year for the education, treatment, rehabilitation and research aspects of the campaign. It will also be spending substantially increased amounts on strengthening law enforcement. Of the $20 million, which will be indexed, $8 million will be allocated for national projects which will be fully funded by the Commonwealth. The remaining $12 million will be available to the States and Territories to match increased expenditure undertaken by them.

The Campaign will be co-ordinated and oversighted by the Ministerial Council on Drug Strategy which will report to the Premiers' Conference. The Council will have the authority to deal with all matters related to drugs of dependence.

The Conference agreed on the introduction of a number of specific initiatives.

Education programs
The Conference agreed that, in consultation with the States:

The National Drug Education Program will be upgraded.
New drug education materials are to be developed, to assist those who

educate, counsel or work with young people and others at risk; materials will be made available for use in schools.

Use will be made of media campaigns, in conjunction with other drug education initiatives, to inform and educate the community about drug problems, and to provide positive directions to assist the community in preventing and overcoming such problems.

Training programs on drug abuse matters for both lay and professional workers in education, health and welfare areas will be improved.

Twenty-four-hour telephone information services on drugs, staffed by trained counsellors, are recommended in those States and Territories where they do not already exist.

Treatment and rehabilitation

The Conference agreed that existing methadone maintenance programs should be expanded and new ones established; the existing guidelines for the use of methadone will be reviewed. The Conference was opposed to the provision of heroin as a treatment for drug addiction.

It was also agreed that a range of special treatment and rehabilitation services for drug abusers be established in teaching hospitals and other major hospitals.

Treatment and rehabilitation services are to be made available to drug-dependent prisoners.

Regular evaluation of programs by community agencies will be a condition of continued government funding of services.

Research and information

The Conference endorsed the establishment of National and State drug data collection systems.

It was agreed that there is a need for more research into the prevention and treatment of drug abuse; it has been agreed in principle that one or more centres of excellence will be established; the States have been invited to bring forward proposals.

Legislation

It was agreed in principle that there should be uniformity of approach among jurisdictions on legislation governing drugs of dependence, and broad consistency on key issues such as classification of drugs and thrust of offences and penalties. The Conference noted that the Commonwealth is developing a model legislation package covering the regulation of the manufacture, distribution and medical use of drugs of dependence; diversion for treatment; and penal provisions. The package will be developed in consultation with the States.

The Conference agreed in principle that legislation be introduced to enable the forfeiture and confiscation of assets of convicted drug dealers.

This matter is to be discussed further by the Standing Committee of Attorneys-General.

The Conference agreed that there should be a review of the controls on the use of barbiturates and it was agreed that this matter be examined urgently. Existing controls on cannabis are to be maintained.

Law enforcement

The Conference endorsed the importance of achieving full co-operation between law enforcement authorities both within jurisdictions and between jurisdictions. The Conference called on all relevant authorities to ensure that they work together in a co-operative way.

The Conference noted the actions being taken by the Commonwealth and the States to strengthen their capabilities to deal with drug trafficking. The Commonwealth will over the next three years be spending $7 million on computer capacity and $10 million on additional manpower for the Australian Federal Police.

It will provide additional resources of the order of $1.5 million over the next two years to enhance the capacity of the Australian Bureau of Criminal Intelligence to provide drugs intelligence to all participating law enforcement agencies.

The Commonwealth will also provide substantial resources—equipment and staff costing $5.5 million over 2 years—to strengthen the capacity of the Australian Customs Service to interdict drugs entering Australia. Fixed barrier operations will be buttressed with additional surveillance, enhanced communication and x-ray machines. There will also be a revised Customs strategy for the North.

The Conference noted that the Australian Police Ministers' Council and the Australian Transport Advisory Council would be considering measures to upgrade waterfront security, including a recommendation for a new National Port Security Authority.

The Conference also noted the recently introduced arrangements for coastal surveillance, including the Coastal Protection Unit within the Australian Federal Police. The importance of ensuring adequate surveillance of the Australian coastline was recognised.

Australia's strong commitment to international efforts to combat drug trafficking will continue. Opportunities for increased co-operation with other countries on narcotics matters will be actively pursued.

The Conference agreed that telephone interception powers can be a valuable aid in investigation of drug trafficking. The Commonwealth will extend such powers in relation to drug trafficking to the States, subject to stringent controls being exercised over their use. The controls will include a requirement for judicial warrants.

The Commonwealth will create a new offence of sending illicit drugs through the mail. The AFP will have powers to examine suspected mail.

The Commonwealth has decided in principle to amend the Customs Act to clarify powers to detain and search persons concealing drugs internally to bring them into Australia; the emphasis will be on detention with medical search as a last resort.

WHO recommendations
The Conference agreed to refer to the Health Ministers' Conference, for consideration without specific endorsement, strategies on alcohol and tobacco as recommended by the World Health Organization.

Drugs and driving
The Conference agreed that States should give consideration to the introduction of zero or equivalent blood alcohol levels for novice drivers, stringent application of penalties, and more severe penalties for persistent drink driving offenders.

Strategy document
The Conference agreed that a document setting out the aims and strategy of the National Campaign Against Drug Abuse should be prepared by the Commonwealth, in consultation with the States, for release as soon as possible.

12
A National Repertoire Of Action Plans

Patterns of action

The step forward into action has been taken; promises for a National Campaign have been made. It is clearly an ambitious Campaign, as can be seen from the recommendations proffered by national interest groups, and accepted by the government, presented in detail in the appendixes to Chapter 11. We have a theme for the Campaign, reduction of the use of legal and control of the use of illegal drugs. It is clearly a truly National Campaign in that all States and all elements of the community will be involved. We know that money is available, and is to be spent on programs and resources in the areas of education, treatment and rehabilitation, research and information, legislation and law enforcement. The co-operation of the community is also to be sought.

But where do we stand, nationally, in terms of resources and programs? We know from Part 2 on strategies in the area that there has been a National Drug Education Program for the last ten years, that treatment and rehabilitation facilities are regarded as overused and under-resourced, that there are no central research or information facilities, that professional education for the health, medical, welfare and teaching professions hardly touches on drug abuse, and that though community development is the preferred method for coping with the effects of social change, including drug abuse, agreement on how community development should be carried out is in its infancy. Is the situation really as black as this?

Does the National Campaign have to start from scratch, except for some experience gained in education?

One way to find the answer is to survey the programs, projects and resources in existence in Australia, and find out from the ground up, what methods are being used, what evaluations have been done, and so diagnose what remains to be done in the way of prevention. This we have attempted to do. Several difficulties became apparent at the outset. Without a central drug information service, or even a recognised centre of research on drugs, there is no clearing house or central point which could act as a check that we had really, or even nearly, found all the resources available. Further, in terms of evaluated, and so reliably recommended, programs there is nearly nothing at all. Most programs have been mounted with insufficient time or resources to allocate to evaluation, and with considerable pressure to 'get on with it' and deliver their services.

On the positive side, there have been a very great number of programs, many receiving the highest informal praise from their clients, and many still going in spite of years of hardship. We were able, without difficulty, to find upwards of sixty such enterprises, some national, some local, some short, some long-term. Since there is no central registry we must simply apologise to those we did not discover. We are well aware that some of the most effective services are delivered by staff so committed and so busy that they have not time to report or to write about their service—and so we could not report on it either. We have heard informally of much excellent work done by individuals and teams, for which there is neither official recognition nor official records. The most important money spent in the National Campaign may well be that spent on helping such services with their reports and evaluations, so that their work is available to others.

In looking for resources, our most valuable single resource was the library of the Alcohol and Drug Foundation, Australia, with Barbara Allan at its head. From there we radiated out like detectives, and the rest of this chapter contains what we found. In terms of the decisions for action from the Drug Summit, the pattern of the resources we found was most interesting. There were a very large number of drug-related enterprises in the treatment field, but these were seldom evaluated, and seldom listed their educational or rehabilitation components; in other words the preventive aspects were rarely emphasised. A short list of treatment services is consequently listed alphabetically in Section E as valuable resources, but without any details.

We had a problem too so far as control measures were concerned. Law libraries full of statutes on rights to personal freedom, and the limitations on those freedoms under certain conditions, did not give us access to any body of law on drugs per se. Jurisprudence does not seem to have tackled this potentially rich field and there was almost no recognition of either law or corrective services as rehabilitation measures. Day by day magistrates courts are setting precedents for the treatment of drug-related offences, but there is little collected wisdom on these trends.

The upwards of sixty effective programs which we mentioned earlier fell naturally into four groups: community action (which included media campaigns); youth and school programs; skills training; and resources and research. There was considerable overlap between these categories, not surprisingly, since in Part 2 we suggested that any effective preventive program would have strong educational and community development elements.

Programs, projects and resources

Before proceeding to describe the actions on drug abuse prevention in Australia, it will be useful to clarify some terms. Projects, programs, services and resources are variously labelled, and we have tried to use the terms consistently throughout. The criteria we established for ourselves were as follows.

(a) A program, we decided, would be a connected series of events, with a coherent thread, a beginning, a middle and an end. A program would usually be described or packaged so that it could be reproduced elsewhere. In a comprehensive program one would expect a pilot or feasibility study, aims and objectives, a description of processes as well as content, a profile of the clients, and some sort of evaluation. Examples of programs could be curriculum designs for schools such as the 'Why Smoke?' program from Sydney, or a media campaign linked to community follow-through, such as the Healthy Lifestyle Program in northern New South Wales.

(b) A project we have kept as a descriptive term for a limited one-off event, with a finite time-span and fixed resources. A pilot, a trial, a short-term intervention, or an intervention appropriate for one time, group or place would be a project. Projects often meet emergency needs, and often turn out to be most effective and models for later programs. DA:NA would be labelled a project, as would a short-burst media campaign.

(c) A resource is usually a fixed service, which can be used to further some more complex objective. Information in print, film, video, poster, pamphlet or spoken form would be a resource, as would a place to meet, a telephone answering or secretarial service, or an emergency referral number. A person can be a resource, as can a place, or even time. Life Education Centres are resources, rather than programs.

(d) A service is supplied whenever there is a process that delivers resources to clients or customers. A service is usually delivered by people, and taken to, or provided for, the convenience of clients. There is clearly overlap, but a curriculum advisory service for teachers would be a service, rather than a resource or a program, as would a telephone counselling facility.

With this clarification, we will proceed to comment on types of drug abuse prevention programs, projects, resources and services available in Australia at the time of DA:NA. Central DA:NA recommendations are given as a focus for the activities listed in each section; the full list of DA:NA recommendations is in Chapter 11, Appendix 1(a).

A. Community

DA:NA recommendations
Community development strategies should be developed and implemented, in order to improve and/or change the social environment which promotes and reinforces drug-taking behaviour.

Since families have an important role in the prevention, early detection and treatment of drug abuse, they should be enabled to fulfil this role by:

> the provision of easily available and relevant information through health services, educational institutions and other appropriate outlets

> access to workers trained to provide family therapy in relation to drugs

recognition of the contribution that can be made by self-help groups of family members to the prevention of emotional and physical trauma and to public education on drugs

encouragement of formation of self-help groups in local areas.

1. Queensland Hotel Patron Care Program

The program began in 1981 and is a joint initiative of Alcohol and Drug Dependence Service and hoteliers. It seeks to encourage, by co-operative development, the promotion of management and marketing practices by the industry that enhance our lifestyle. This includes enjoyment of alcohol by those who choose it, in pleasant surroundings, where social cohesion rather than social isolation is fostered. Other services such as good food, entertainment and non-alcoholic drinks are available. The outcome is hoped to be a reduction in the incidence and prevalence of alcohol problems in our society.

Contact: Alcohol and Drug Dependence Service, Queensland
Ph. (07) 2296566

2. Lions/ADFA Foundation—National

This co-ordinating body was formed in 1984 to promote better involvement of service clubs in the vital area of community drug education.

In South Australia for example, the Lions Clubs conduct a smorgasbord of drug education programs which takes two different approaches, 'Do it yourself' programs for clubs and organisations (with a bit of help from Lions staff) or drug education programs for community groups. Lions staff receive input from DASC (Drug and Alcohol Services Council) and all programs are evaluated by DASC.

Contact: Drug and Alcohol Services Council, South Australia
Ph. (08) 2726144
Contact ADFA for general information on the Foundation.

3. Pharmacists' Community Health Education Campaign—New South Wales

The campaign, launched in 1984, was prepared by the Pharmacy Guild of Australia. A new slogan has been adopted, 'the chemist is your first aid', which is intended to sum up the message to the community that pharmacists are health advisers, the immediate point of contact for many people. A major part of the campaign is the production of education material for use in schools at upper and lower secondary levels. Prepared with the assistance of the New South Wales Department of Health, teachers kits have been produced which include a series of lectures and project material on health and health care services, the history and development of medicines, safe use of medicines, etc.

The other facet of the campaign is the regular publication of *Health facts*, a newsletter which the Guild is making available free.

Contact: Pharmacy Guild—New South Wales Branch
Ph. (02) 4383333

4. Pregnant Pause campaign

The Pregnant Pause campaign was conducted in Newcastle in 1980-81. It was a pilot health promotion/intervention program to reduce inappropriate drug use during pregnancy. The campaign comprised a mass media campaign, a community education program involving group discussions with unions, service clubs, nursing mothers groups, parent and citizen groups and technical college students, a professional education program for health personnel and support services for the pregnant woman.

Results from the campaign suggest that pregnant women do want drug use information, and that the existing pre-natal care system is the best system through which to provide it.

The Pregnant Pause project has been adopted by other States throughout Australia.

Contact: Drug and Alcohol Authority, New South Wales
Ph. (02) 2176163

5. Alcohol and Drug Education in Aboriginal and Islander Communities—Queensland

The project undertakes to examine the patterns of use, attitudes to and problems associated with alcohol and other drugs which are unique to Aboriginal communities, and to develop educational programs and resources for primary and secondary schools in Aboriginal communities which relate to the specific interests, concerns and needs of the people in those communities.

The guiding principle of the project is that the Aboriginal community will be involved considerably from the outset in the planning, trialling and implementing of resources and strategies designed, rather than being simply the recipient of programs designed from without and imposed on it.

Contact: Alcohol and Drug Programs Unit, Department of Education—Queensland
Ph. (07) 2247189

6. National Alcohol and Drug Dependence Industry Program (NADDIP)

The program aims to identify, as early as possible, all persons suffering from alcohol and/or other drug problems, as indicated by falling standards of work performance; to motivate all persons with alcohol and/or other drug-related problems to seek treatment or other assistance; to assist all persons within the work environment to develop responsible attitudes towards alcohol and other drugs. In recent years the program has broadened to assist employees with non-drug personal problems.

There are offices in all States and Territories and program coverage has reached about seven per cent of the Australian workforce, via approximately six hundred specific contacts with work places, e.g. Commonwealth Public Service, unions, hospitals, educational institutions, businesses (large and small) and the armed services.

The program is funded by the Department of Health under a Community Health Services Grant to the Alcohol and Drug Foundation, Australia.

Contact: Alcohol and Drug Foundation, Australia, Canberra City
Ph. (062) 473939

7. Community Approach to Drug Abuse Prevention Project (CADAP)—National

This is a project of the Alcohol and Drug Foundation, Australia supported by the Commonwealth Department of Health, National Community Health Program, and co-ordinated by a team based in Canberra. The project aims to assist community groups throughout Australia who are concerned about drug abuse in their area and to help them to help themselves, that is, to prevent such problems from occurring in the future. Communities are encouraged to examine the reasons for their problems, to work out their own solutions and to be actively involved in improving the circumstances in which they live.

Contact: CADAP, Belconnen, Canberra
Ph. (062) 513222

8. Drink driving publicity programs—Western Australia
In 1983-84 a major State-wide drink driving program was initiated, supported by locally produced television and radio commercials based on the colloquial expression 'How ya doing, mate?' To maintain the momentum, the National Safety Council (NSC) of Western Australia in 1985 continued its program with the theme 'Plan alternatives to driving after drinking'.

Contact: National Safety Council of Western Australia
Ph. (09) 2721666

See also 'Drink driving campaigns' in Section F, 'Media'.

9. North Coast Healthy Lifestyle Program—New South Wales
This program used media as part of its approach to positively influence behaviour presumed to be associated with a healthy lifestyle. It focused on eating, fitness, smoking and drinking. TV advertisements, radio, pamphlets and press coverage were all used to get the health messages across to the public and to encourage people to contact the health agency staff who were geared to provide a variety of services and other activities. The approach took into account peer pressure, commercial advertising techniques, emotional appeal and humour. Although this project is now completed the literature is still readily available and of considerable value in planning lifestyle programs.

Contact: Drug and Alcohol Authority, New South Wales
Ph. (02) 2176163

10. Operation Oldies—National
This links the isolated elderly in the community with high school students. It was initiated in Canberra in 1979 by Judy Cole after a group of health professionals expressed concern for elderly

patients requesting medication for depression and insomnia. The aim of the program is to ease the isolation of these older people by establishing a one to one relationship with a student. The expectation is that a long-term friendship will result with benefit to both participants.

A training manual is now available and is a useful resource for schools and community groups wishing to become involved in such a program.

Contact: Health Promotion Branch, ACT Health Authority, PO Box 825, Canberra City, 2601
Ph. (062) 454537

11. Billboard Utilising Graffitists Against Unhealthy Promotions (BUGA-UP)

BUGA-UP used spray cans of paint to 'reface' billboards which carry advertising for products such as tobacco and alcohol. BUGA-UP used this method to expose the devices the advertisers are using —demystifying their process.

Members of BUGA-UP have been charged in New South Wales magistrates courts, and released as having provided information in the public interest.

Contact: MOP-UP (Movement Opposed to the Promotion of Unhealthy Products), PO Box 47, Clifton Hill, 3068

12. Woma Committee—South Australia

Woma is a co-ordinated committee for Aboriginal alcohol and drug services throughout South Australia. The objective is to assist community groups or individuals to develop their own projects. This committee also represents various issues on Aboriginal alcohol and drug problems.

Contact: Woma Committee, 121 Wright Street, Adelaide
Ph. (08) 2118055

B. Youth and schools

DA:NA recommendations
Education, at all levels, should include programs which prepare people to make more informed decisions about lifestyle (e.g.

problem solving, decision making) and should be part of the standard curriculum.

Education programs about drugs and their social setting should permeate the whole educational process, including the education of professional people [health and welfare personnel, teachers, medical practitioners, etc.].

Parental involvement (where appropriate) needs to be considered.

1. *National Drug Education Program (NDEP)*
This program has been funded by the Commonwealth Government since it began in 1970-71. The NDEP aims to assist people, particularly the young, to make informed, responsible decisions about drug use. Commonwealth funds have been used to provide resource people and resource material as a stimulus for the development of actual programs in schools and communities. A national committee has developed guidelines for drug education programs.

Details of objectives can be found in Chapter 8, and many of the school programs listed here have been funded by NDEP (now supervised by the National Drug Education Committee—NDEC).

Contact: Drug Dependence Branch, Commonwealth Department of Health
Ph. (062) 891555

2. *Youth Life Project—New South Wales*
This is a response to a need for health promotion programs designed by and for young people. Ten young people (funded) are trained by health professionals, and the group then develops health promotion and drama action programs to present to local youth centres, youth support schemes and schools. Major goals are to encourage young people to actively participate in their own health promotion.

Contact: Adolescent Medical Unit, Camperdown, Sydney
Ph. (02) 6926446

3. *Why Smoke?—New South Wales*
A comprehensive kit for schools with teacher's manual, training program for teachers and parents, and classroom materials. The kit

was developed in the Western Metropolitan Health Region of NSW and has been used widely in NSW and ACT schools.

Contact: Drug and Alcohol Authority, New South Wales
Ph. (02) 2176163

4. Education about Drugs: K-10—Northern Territory

A resource manual for teachers, designed to assist them in the classroom in identifying important issues for each year level (K-year 10), it contains ideas considered important to be raised with students to assist them in making responsible decisions about drugs. In-service courses are made available in skills training to assist teachers to implement this program. It is currently in operation throughout Northern Territory schools and is being evaluated.

Contact: Department of Education, Northern Territory
Ph. (089) 804211

5. Drug Education for Apprentices in the Wood Trade—South Australia

This drug education program is organised through the TAFE colleges for apprentice students, and the emphasis is on prevention and primary intervention.

Contact: Drug and Alcohol Services Council, South Australia
Ph. (08) 2726144

6. Belconnen Care Education—ACT

This school-based curriculum development project (years 7-10), initiated and developed by the whole school community (parents, teachers and students), aims to provide a caring and harmonious environment in which the social and emotional needs of the students can be met. A blueprint for teachers and parents for creating the right climate for the construction and maintenance of a range of personal attributes and skills in each student, the program commences with an in-service training course for group leaders and includes topics such as drug education, communication skills, sex education and health development.

Contact: Alcohol and Drug Service, ACT Health Authority,
PO Box 825, Canberra City, 2601
Ph. (062) 451111

7. Peer Support Foundation—New South Wales

The Peer Support Program (PSP) utilises students as an existing communication resource in schools. Based on the principle that people absorb information and values from each other, PSP develops caring feelings in the school community and reinforces the school environment by providing more personal contact between young and older students. PSP was initiated by Elizabeth Campbell in 1971 at a school when a 16-year-old boy had died of a heroin overdose. Since then, the program has been introduced into high schools throughout New South Wales with great success. Several schools have integrated the program into the school curriculum. PSP is supported by public subscriptions and service clubs.

Contact: The Peer Support Foundation Limited
Ph. (02) 9775022

8. Life Education Centre (LEC)—New South Wales

LEC is a drug education program which aims to explain to children the intricate workings of the human body and the way in which different substances can affect the delicate equilibrium of its systems. LEC is a classroom of the twenty-first century which is equipped with electronic aids, sophisticated sight and sound techniques and electronic modules. Children from 4 to 11 years attend the centre each year and move through an education program to suit their age group. Children and teachers are given book material for continuing studies in the care of the human body.

LEC of the Wayside Chapel in Kings Cross was started by the Reverend Ted Noffs in 1979.

Evaluation questionnaires are completed by teachers and pupils on the presentation (and not the achievement) of the overall program aims and objectives. The New South Wales Drug and Alcohol Authority are currently evaluating the program.

Contact: Life Education Centre
Ph. (02) 3586577

9. Teenagers, Alcohol and Road Safety—Victoria

A program for schools which consists of a set of teaching materials targeted for secondary students in years 8-10, it comprises a series of twenty-one suggested lesson segments, each with teachers' notes and students' worksheets. The materials promote the teaching of values and clarification of issues through discussion and role play; they aim to provide factual content to dispel common myths about alcohol and they consider individuals, parental values and peer group pressures and the need for making independent choices about behaviour and attitudes. Ninety per cent of schools in Victoria are currently using the materials. In 1983 a control group was part of an evaluation of this program.

Contact: Road Traffic Authority, Road Safety and Traffic Bureau
Ph. (03) 8102666

10. Drink Driving Education Materials Project—New South Wales
This is a joint project by the New South Wales Department of Education and the New South Wales Traffic Authority in response to the increasing involvement of young drivers in drink-driving fatalities. The program consists of drink-driving education material for secondary schools and an in-service education course to introduce the resource materials to teachers.

The program was evaluated in 1982 to determine whether changes occurred in knowledge and attitude as a result of exposure to drink driving materials.

Contact: Traffic Authority, Road Safety and Traffic Bureau
Ph. (02) 6638246

11. Schools Program of the Smoking and Health Project—Western Australia
The schools program is primarily handled by trained teachers in a co-ordinated effort between the Smoking and Health Project and the Education Project and is one segment of the three-year campaign designed to reduce the incidence of smoking in Western Australia. Schools have been provided with a year 7 smoking prevention program designed to make children aware of the short-term effects of smoking on the body as well as encouraging them to develop strategies to refuse a cigarette if offered.

In addition a smoking education resource manual for teachers at either junior, middle, upper primary or high school levels is available. This provides a series of activities from which teachers may design their own program or unit of work. It also contains a comprehensive resource list of all available smoking education material in Western Australia. The resource material was piloted in schools in 1983.

Contact: Co-ordinator of Schools and Youth Programs,
Smoking and Health Project Team,
514 Hay Street, Perth

12. Smoking Education Project—Queensland
The major aim of the program is to reduce the rate of recruitment to smoking. Secondary aims are to develop responsible smoking attitudes and behaviours and to assist students who wish to quit. The program revolves around a teachers handbook and activity-based students workbook. The activities allow the students to individually work through the book clarifying their values in relation to smoking, seeking information and making a decision whether they want to be a smoker or non-smoker. The role of the teacher is that of a facilitator and they are encouraged to be non-moralistic and non-judgmental. The evaluation showed that the main aim of reducing recruitment to smoking had been achieved.

Contact: Smoking Education Consultant
Ph. (07) 2247784

13. 'Hooked on Health' Week at Enmore High School—New South Wales
A healthy lifestyle week was organised for year 8 at Enmore High School in response to increasing solvent abuse by some of the young people attending the school; the week was named Hooked on Health by the students. Health workers, youth workers and teachers planned, implemented and evaluated the program. During the week, staff from Newtown Community Care Centre, Careforce and Adolescent Medical Unit went to Enmore High to run workshops on stress management and relaxation, dangers of tobacco, alcohol and solvent sniffing, posture and back care, nutrition, inter-personal communication skills, youth culture and leisure. The program reached 140 young people.

Contact: Royal Alexander Hospital for Children, Adolescent
Medical Unit, Camperdown, Sydney
Ph. (02) 6926556

14. Student Council Stop Smoking Project—ACT

As part of International Youth Year the co-ordinating committee for Stop Smoking Activities in the ACT set up an integrated project involved with the CADAP team, ACT Health Promotion Branch and Alcohol and Drug Service. Each high school student representative council was asked to nominate a team of five students. Each school team over a period of three days works on an action plan to reduce the incidence of smoking in their respective schools. The plan is then put into effect by the student council, and will be evaluated by the ACT Health Authority.

Contact: Health Promotion Branch (Youth and Schools Section), ACT Health Authority, PO Box 825, Canberra City, 2601 Ph. (062) 454537

15. Street Leaders Camp—Northern Territory

The program is aimed at street bush leaders in Alice Springs. A five-day youth camp for identified leaders of glue- and petrol-inhaling activity is conducted to introduce leadership styles, and to educate participants towards adopting an inhalant-free lifestyle.

Contact: Drug and Alcohol Bureau, Northern Territory

16. Alcohol: Its Science and Sociology—South Australia

An alcohol program has been incorporated into the existing South Australian science syllabus. The program has nine units. Examples of the topics covered are: history and geography of winemaking, botany of alcohol, horticulture and propagation, effects on the body, psychology of drink. Activities include experiments, discussion questions and debates, films and posters. This program has been evaluated by its author, Hewitson, and according to his research the program appears to prevent alcohol abuse, without having any impact on long-established abusers. Recent heavy drinkers seem to modify their behaviour and the results suggest that the program should be introduced at an age before regular abuse has started, viz. end of year 8 or beginning of year 9.

Contact: M. Hewitson, Salisbury Education Centre, Salisbury, South Australia

17. A School-based Curriculum in Health and Physical Development for Years K-12

Contact: The Woy Woy Cluster Group of Schools, North Sydney Region In-Service Education

18. Body Owners' Program

This is an imaginative and amusing program for children in primary schools, which includes an exercise program and dietary information. Trialled in South Australia in the late seventies and thoroughly evaluated, it was found to produce increased alertness and more involvement in school-related tasks. The delightful *Body owners' manual* was created for the program and is distributed through bookshops.

Contact: Dr Tony Worsley and Dr Katherine Baghurst, CSIRO Division of Human Nutrition, Adelaide

Overseas school-based programs

The following programs (information provided by Centre for Education and Information on Drugs and Alcohol, CEIDA) have proved of value in countries with a similar educational tradition to Australia's. Such programs will need, of course, trialling and amending for another country, but they provide valuable source material.

19. All about me—England

A set of booklets entitled *All about me* are a guide for teachers in infant and lower primary schools (years 5-8), offering practical suggestions and teaching strategies for work in health education. Topics covered are: finding out about myself, how did I begin?, what is growing?, what helps me grow?, looking after myself, keeping safe, and knowing about others.

Contact: Schools Council Project, Essex, England

20. Think well—England

A set of booklets entitled *Think well* form a teachers guide for the middle years of schooling (9-13). Topics covered include: my self, one of many, from sickness to health?, deadly decisions, time to spare, food for thought, get clean!, skills and spills (safety).

Contact: *Think well*, Thomas Nelson and Sons Ltd, London

21. Alcohol Education—Ten lesson plans for grades 7 and 8; Ten lesson plans for grades 9 and 10—Canada
This set of ten lesson plans, each dealing with aspects of alcohol use, was developed and field tested in co-operation with the Toronto Board of Education. The lesson plans were developed to provide the teacher with as much information concerning alcohol and the process of teaching about alcohol as is both possible and reasonable. The lessons were presented merely as a foundation upon which teachers could build their own programs.

For grades 7 and 8, topics covered include: alcohol and myths, advertising, why people drink, effects of drinking, positive uses of alcohol, drinking and driving, teenagers and alcohol, alcohol and the family, alcohol and athletics, student research and consolidation.

For grades 9 and 10, topics include: alcohol and myths, media, needs, youth, the law, driving, alcohol campaign, the family, fitness, sexuality.

Contact: Addiction Research Foundation of Ontario, Canada and the Toronto Board of Education

22. Decision-making Skills about Legal and Illegal Drugs—England
A six-ten hour prototype of a situational or decision-making approach to drug education was trialled by teachers in English and Danish schools and was found to be fairly effective in increasing knowledge and in teaching decision-making skills to fourth formers. It is based on the premise that education has to be made relevant to students' future lives by dealing with facts about legal and illegal drugs and exploring students' feelings about drugs and about themselves. It places discussion of facts and feelings within the context of the social situations in which they will be used.

Contact: ISDD (Institute for the Study of Drug Dependence), Health Education Council, England

23. Westchester County Student Assistance Program—USA

The Student Assistance Program developed in Westchester County, New York is based on an employee assistance program model, and uses professional counsellors to provide alcohol and drug abuse intervention and prevention services for high school students who have alcoholic parents, have been abusing alcohol or drugs, and/or exhibit behavioural and academic problems or are experiencing stress that could be related to parental or student alcohol or other drug abuse. Initially implemented in six high schools through funding provided by the New York Division of Alcoholism and Alcohol Abuse, this program had been implemented in twenty-two schools as of September 1982. It provides four types of early intervention, including: group counselling sessions for students with alcoholic parents; individual, family, or group counselling services for students who are using alcohol or drugs dysfunctionally; counselling services for students who exhibit poor school performance; working with parent and community groups to develop different ways of handling problems related to adolescent alcohol and drug abuse.

Contact: Ellen Morehouse, Westchester County Department of Community Mental Health, 148 Martine Avenue, White Plains, New York
Ph. (914) 6822699

24. Natural Helpers Program—USA

Within every school an informal 'helping network' exists. The Natural Helpers Program is based on this simple premise. Students with problems naturally seek out other students—and occasionally teachers or other school staff. Because they trust them, they ask them for advice, for help in getting assistance or just to provide sympathetic listening. The Natural Helpers Program utilises Natural Helpers who include a cross-section of students and adult staff members, identified and selected through an anonymous school-wide survey. After they are identified, they are invited to participate in the Natural Helpers Program and receive at least thirty hours of training in communication skills so they can listen empathetically and help others. They also receive information on local resources and training on identifying their own limits in order to make referrals when necessary. They are not professionally trained therapists or counsellors.

Contact: Carol Mooney, Roberts and Associates,
9131 California Avenue, S.W., Seattle,
Washington, 98136
Ph. (206) 9328409

25. Here's Looking at You, Two—USA
This is a comprehensive school curriculum for grades K-12, which can be taught as a unit or integrated into a variety of areas. A teacher training program involves a thirty-hour course to prepare teachers to implement the alcohol and drug curriculum in their classrooms.

Contact: Clay Roberts, Roberts and Associates,
9131 California Avenue, S.W., Seattle,
Washington, 98136
Ph. (206) 9328409

26. CASPAR—USA
This successful program embraces teachers, students, health professionals, and the public. As an outgrowth of the Cambridge-Somerville Mental Health and Retardation community development services, the CASPAR Alcohol Education program began modestly several years ago with a locally funded workshop for school personnel. At the core of CASPAR (Cambridge and Somerville Program for Alcohol Rehabilitation) are twenty-hour small group workshops for hundreds of elementary and secondary teachers, guidance counsellors, and administrators. Initial workshops use games, role playing, discussions and other techniques to help participants evaluate their own feelings, to separate facts from myths on alcohol and alcoholism, and to understand the dynamics of alcoholism as a family illness. An advanced workshop explores effective methods for teaching about alcohol. Experienced workshop participants have devised an original alcohol education curriculum for grades 3 through 12, which has now been field tested with more than fifteen hundred students.

Contact: Lena DiCicco, 226 Highland Avenue, Somerville,
Massachusetts, 02143
Ph. (617) 6232080

27. *Sumner Tobacco and Alcohol Risk Reduction Project, (STARR Project) USA*

The program which they developed was called the Family Interaction Program, which trains parents to conduct prevention activities with their elementary and junior high school age children.

The Family Interaction Program makes use of two basic resource documents: the *Family activity book* and *A leader's guide*. The *Family activity book* contains more than twenty activities and is designed to involve all family members in alcohol and drug education. *A leader's guide* outlines a four-part parent education program designed to help parents learn how to effectively conduct the prevention activities and it also provides step-by-step suggestions about how parents and schools can organise, publicise, and present the parent training program.

Contact: Lynette Benaltabe, 1212 Wood Avenue, Sumner, Washington, 93890
Ph. (206) 8632201

C. Skills training: professionals and community

DA:NA recommendations

Education programs about drugs and their social setting should permeate the whole educational process, including the education of professional people.

Persons or authorities responsible for drug education programs should consult with Education Departments to design learning kits and units of work across the broad range of drug issues.

Special professional training at all levels, including medical schools, is required. In particular:

(a) Professional (postgraduate and continuing) education, related to drugs, including primary prevention, needs to be available and at the highest possible standard for all health, welfare and police and correctional service personnel.
(b) The role of all health and welfare professionals in the process of early identification and intervention needs to be defined and appropriate training given to meet these needs.
(c) Staff involved in the management of all types of drug problems should be enabled to have regular and relevant staff

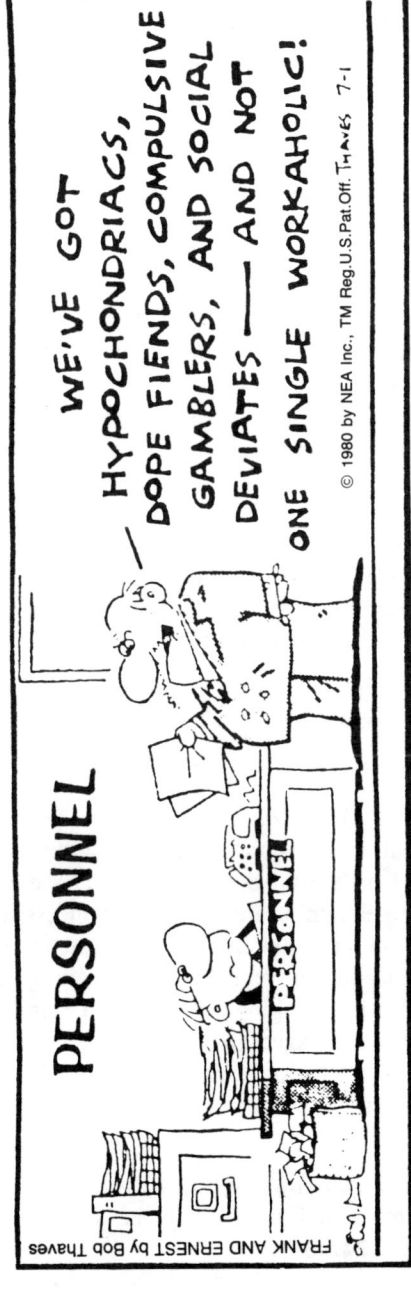

Cartoon by Thaves, reprinted by permission of United Press International on behalf of Newspaper Enterprise Association, from *Australian*, 21 April 1981

development and professional updating through appropriate in-service training, and postgraduate training through special courses should be provided in tertiary institutions with specially dedicated funds.

1. Training courses—New South Wales

Two of the principal functions of the Health Education Unit include consultancy and training for curriculum developers, teachers, parents and others concerned with health and drug education. Three training courses offered in 1985 include:

Program Development Approach to Drug Education—offers teachers, parents and others the opportunity to examine a range of alcohol, tobacco and drug education programs and obtain assistance in planning programs.

Drug Education—Assertiveness Skills Approach—introduces participants to assertiveness skills as a way of helping adolescents to cope with conflict situations they may encounter.

What Parents Need to Know about Drugs—this course offers participants the opportunity to increase their knowledge and understanding of the use and the role of drugs in society today.

Contact: Health Education Unit, Sydney Institute of Education
Ph. (02) 6602855, ext. 212

2. Drug Education Skills Training Seminars—Queensland

Two teachers from each secondary school within an education region are trained at a four-day seminar. The emphasis is on training teachers to design strategies which will assist students to develop personal and inter- personal skills. These include skills for building self-esteem, setting realistic goals, coping with anxiety, effective communicating, making decisions and managing conflict. Teachers are then encouraged to apply these strategies in drug education to their own existing school programs. By mid 1985 one of these seminars will have been conducted for each education region.

Contact: Alcohol and Drug Programs Unit,
Department of Education, Queensland
Ph. (07) 2247189

3. Symposium for Professionals Working with Patients Affected by Drug Misuse—South Australia
A symposium co-sponsored by the South Australian Health Commission and AMSAD aims to address topics including: the use, misuse and abuse of opiates in patients suffering chronic pain and in methadone programs, the early detection of drug and alcohol abuse in general practice and hospitals, confrontation/ management skills in clients with problems of drug and alcohol abuse, drug-seeking behaviour and ways of coping with it, drug abuse in professionals.

Contact: Drug and Alcohol Services Council, South Australia
Ph. (08) 2726144

4. Guidelines and Strategies for Drug Education, Voluntary Alcohol and Drug Agencies and Community Welfare Agencies— Victoria
Many staff of regional agencies are called on to undertake drug education upon request from community groups; in the absence of established principles and strategies for the delivery of such services, their quality varies greatly. This project is designed to develop and pilot a set of coherent policy and procedure guidelines for drug education conducted by voluntary and community welfare agencies.

Contact: Alcohol, Drug and Forensic Branch,
Health Commission of Victoria
Ph. (03) 6167777

5. Australian Medical Society on Alcohol and Drug Related Problems (AMSAD)—National
Its membership is open to all professionals interested and active in the field. Its aim is to improve the competence and to increase the interest in this field of all professionals. It publishes the *Australian alcohol/drug review* twice each year and has a membership of about two hundred.

Primary concern is to increase the level of knowledge and expertise of its own members, and those of the medical profession, and to improve the attitudes of the profession towards the prevention and treatment of alcohol and drug-related problems.

Contact: Drug and Alcohol Authority, New South Wales
Ph. (02) 2176163

6. Medical Education Project—New South Wales

The current Medical Education Project was set up by the New South Wales Department of Health in late 1984 as a result of concern that medical schools were not adequately equipping their students to deal with prevention, detection and rehabilitation in the area of alcohol and other drug problems. It follows the lead taken by the Nurses Education Project which is currently being implemented in nursing schools in New South Wales. The project is attempting to elicit information and opinions on how the present situation can be improved and to develop a plan which will encourage and assist teachers of medicine to include and integrate relevant aspects of the subject into both the compulsory and elective curricula.

The project may be further developed on a national basis.

Contact: Royal Prince Alfred Hospital, Sydney
Ph. (02) 5166111 ext. 8956

7. Professional Training and Development—Western Australia Drug Education Workshops for Teachers

This project involves the development and implementation of a comprehensive information and skills-based approach to training high school teachers in the principles and techniques of drug education. The workshops are conducted in metropolitan and country regions throughout the State and involve teachers from government and non-government schools. The education workshops were evaluated in 1984 to determine their effectiveness in assisting teachers to conduct drug education programs in their schools and to determine the extent to which resource materials were used.

Contact: Alcohol and Drug Authority, Western Australia
Ph. (09) 3212444

8. Counsellor Course for Aboriginal People—Western Australia

The Drug Education Centre in 1985 conducted an intensive six-week Alcohol Counsellor Training Course for Aboriginal people. The first three weeks were devoted to lectures and other formal input and the final three weeks involved placement of course participants with Aboriginal workers at Kulila, the Aboriginal

Medical Service and the Alcohol and Drug Authority.

Contact: Alcohol and Drug Authority, Western Australia
Ph. (09) 3212444

9. Smoking Cessation Program for Use in General Practice
An intervention program was developed in collaboration with general practitioners following a three-year study in which GPs' use of a smoking cessation program was evaluated. The key elements of the intervention program are: patient education relating salivary nicotine and lung function tests to cigarette-related diseases, advice on withdrawal symptoms, weight management, substitutes and alternatives to smoking and follow-up visits to the GP.

A kit titled *Smoke screen—stop smoking* is available for GPs and contains educational material, information for patients and record cards for 100 patients.

Contact: Dr Robyn Richmond, Professor Ian Webster,
School of Community Medicine,
University of New South Wales, Sydney
Ph. (02) 6972512

10. Family Medicine Program—National
Funded from national health promotion funds, the Family Medicine Program is a branch of the Royal Australian College of General Practitioners which provides updating and skills training for both new and experienced general practitioners. Based on problem solving and problem-based learning, the program runs a series of seminars and workshops.

Contact: Family Medicine Program in each Australian capital city.

D. Resources and information

DA:NA recommendations
Reliable information concerning drug use and abuse, including information relevant to the special needs of particular groups and communities, should be readily available.

Research, evaluation and the development of national databases must be an essential part of a national drug policy, both with respect to the development and management of programs and the administration of drug controls.

1. Alcohol and Drug Foundation, Australia Library and Information Service—National

In response to community demands for drug information, and in an effort to counter the duplication of effort and expense, the ADFA library in Canberra has initiated a comprehensive directory on current drug information sources throughout Australia. It is a State by State directory of drug information sources, their strengths and weaknesses, their collection policies and details of service provided. ADFA lists and briefly describes films, kits, pamphlets, posters and major reports.

Contact: Alcohol and Drug Foundation, Australia Library,
GPO Box 477, Canberra City, 2601
Ph. (062) 496888

2. Resource Development—Western Australia

This includes the development of training and reference manuals, information sheets, video material, etc. Specific topics for 1985 include: alcohol and its effect on the body, rehabilitation services in Western Australia, basic concepts booklet, detoxification manual, handbook on the Authority and its services, addiction studies handbook.

Contact: Alcohol and Drug Authority, Western Australia
Ph. (09) 3212444

3. Healthy Lifestyles Promotion—Queensland

To support the Skills Training Program (mentioned in Section C), the Queensland Alcohol and Drug Programs Unit of the Department of Education has produced a series of posters directed to adolescents, promoting a 'drug-free lifestyle', together with a booklet for young people on 'how to say no to drugs'. The theme of the promotion is self-care and personal development within the context of healthy lifestyle, e.g. satisfaction and personal achievements, care of self through exercise, diet and stress management, and communication skills.

Posters, pamphlets, film guides, an alcohol education kit for secondary schools and an activities book for teachers called *Interpersonal skills in drug education* have been produced. Discussion and workshop video cassettes are available: *Best of friends*, aimed at helping secondary students understand the pressures leading to alcohol use and abuse; *B.Y.O.*, on adolescent drinking; *Enough guts to say no*, on adolescent smoking; and *Drinking, driving, surviving.*

Contact: Department of Education, PO Box 33,
North Quay, 4000
Ph. (07) 2247189

4. Health Pamphlets Designed by Youth for Youth—ACT
Secondary students designed, developed and produced a series of health-related pamphlets. Ten Health Promotion staff piloted the fact sheets in two secondary schools. Students were asked to comment on style, content and possible promotion strategies. Their ideas were collated and senior art students from a local college completed the art work, graphics and final products.

Contact: Health Promotion Branch (Youth and Schools Section), ACT Health Authority, PO Box 825,
Canberra City, 2601
Ph. (062) 454537

5. Nurses Education Project—New South Wales
Developed by CEIDA with the assistance of two nurse educators, it includes teaching guidelines and resource material for nurse education, in fourteen teaching modules. The package contains background material and teaching ideas on topics such as community health, nurses and drug use, nursing practice, etc. It was introduced in 1984 and is now used extensively throughout New South Wales.

Contact: Centre for Education and Information on Drugs and Alcohol, Surry Hills
Ph. (02) 3312196

6. Free to Choose—South Australia
This program, published in 1984, was adapted from TACADE (Teachers Advisory Council on Alcohol and Drug Education, United Kingdom), and is an instruction package for secondary teachers designed by the Drug and Alcohol Services Council to help young people make better choices in possible drug use.

Contact: Health Education Advisers, Wattle Park Teachers Centre, Adelaide
Ph. (08) 3324555

7. Health education news and views—Western Australia

Journals relevant to health education are scanned and reviewed by Health Education staff on a regular basis to provide health professionals with up-to-date information relevant to drug education. Abstracts are prepared and included in a quarterly publication. Two recent special editions focused on alcohol and tobacco smoking.

Contact: Health Promotion Service, Perth
Ph. (09) 3280241 ext. 516

8. Substance Abuse Monthly (SAM)

SAM is a regular update of current information and recent research in the field of alcohol and other drug use and abuse. It is essentially a survey of the current literature. While clinical and experimental data are not excluded, SAM focuses on the psychological aspects of drug use and abuse. A wide range of journals is scanned but only those articles with direct application to the field of substance abuse are abstracted.

Contact: Alcohol, Drug and Forensic Branch,
Mental Health Division,
Health Commission of Victoria
Ph. (03) 6168024

9. Resource Development—Western Australia

The Western Australian Alcohol and Drug Authority has expanded its education section resource base and developed training and reference manuals, information sheets and video materials. Specific topics for development during 1985 include videos for Aborigines, alcohol and its effect on the body, rehabilitation services in Western Australia and a detoxification manual.

Contact: Alcohol and Drug Authority, Western Australia
Ph. (09) 3212444

10. Solvent Abuse Education Program—Western Australia

The objective of the program is to increase awareness amongst health workers and educators about the problems of solvent abuse and the way in which this issue (including petrol sniffing) can be handled. In 1983 a leaflet covering the issue was prepared and it has been reprinted by the Health Promotion Service and the Western Australian Alcohol and Drug Authority. This information has been sent to medical practitioners and health workers throughout the State. It is proposed that Health Promotion staff will conduct workshops and speak at regional meetings of community health workers on the problems of solvent abuse.

Contact: Alcohol and Drug Authority, Western Australia
Ph. (09) 3212444

11. Australian Sports Medicine Federation
ASMF have developed a drug education resource package aimed at all groups involved in sport, including children and parents. The resource material outlines the short- and long-term effects of drug use by sports participants, including tobacco smoking, alcohol and caffeine consumption.

Contact: Australian Sports Medicine Federation,
Drugs in Sport Co-ordinator, Canberra
Ph. (062) 950032

12. Pallister House—New South Wales
This is a major resource centre for health education, including drug education, for New South Wales. The health education centre for the Northern Metropolitan Region of the New South Wales Health Commission, it sells and leases videotapes, audiotapes and booklets and provides consultation programs and courses.

Contact: Pallister House,
Health, Media and Information Centre,
North Sydney
Ph. (02) 4394288

E. Treatment and rehabilitation centres

DA:NA recommendations
Programs for drug users should be accredited and the guidelines for accreditation should include levels of care such as:

(a) A person considered for inclusion in any treatment program should have access to full information and counselling about the nature of the program.

(b) Where any person requires admission into a treatment program she/he has a right to well-maintained clinics and rehabilitation services, and access twenty-four hours a day to a counselling service and crisis intervention.
(c) A wide range of interventions aimed at assisting individuals manifesting harmful drug behaviours should be provided.
(d) Community programs should be part of the community, staffed by community members and legitimised by involvement of local community leaders.

1. General treatment/rehabilitation centres
These centres, with some variation, treat all ages and sexes and drug problems and are run for inpatients and/or outpatients. They offer a variety of detoxification, medical care, counselling, education and training services. Some are based in hospitals or health centres while others are run independently by both government and private agencies. Some also work on public education and research. Examples are:

Aborigines and Islanders Alcohol Relief Service, Cairns—(070) 512910
Banyan House, Darwin—(089) 852479
Bourke St Drug Advisory Centre, Sydney—(02) 6607863
Lantadd, Launceston—(003) 313944
Mancare Community, Canberra—(062) 951256
Moreland Hall, Melbourne—(03) 3862876
Quo Vadis, Byford, Western Australia—(095) 231572

2. More specific approaches
Quit Smoking Programs (e.g. Fresh Start, Victoria; Quit. For Life, New South Wales—see Section F) have been run all over Australia by the State Health Authorities and Cancer Councils and offer or refer on to a variety of assistance such as individual counselling, group therapy, hypnotherapy, acupuncture.

Some services such as Odyssey House are run as therapeutic communities on a very structural prescriptive model.

Alcoholics Anonymous and Narcotics Anonymous are self-help organisations in which previously dependent people support each other to keep up their drug-free lifestyle.

Alateen is a self-help recovery program with emphasis on teenagers and their problems. The program offers hope, encouragement and emotional support to families and friends of alcoholics. It is a worldwide fellowship similar to Al-Anon, offering twenty-four hour service.

Contact: Al-Anon Family Group, Australia General Services, GPO Box 1002, Melbourne.
Sydney, ph. (02) 6731638

3. Specialised targets
Family Living, Adelaide is fully residential and offers treatment and rehabilitation for drug-dependent people and their families—(08) 423422.

Phoebe House, Sydney assists heroin-dependent mothers with young children in a methadone program and to develop parenting skills—(02) 6607863.

Drugs in the Family, Canberra is a support group for the families of (largely heroin) dependent people. Weekly meetings are held which provide education and mutual support—(062) 451836.

F. Media

DA:NA recommendations
Media campaigns play an important part in public health. They must be directed at well-identified target groups and have clear objectives. This Workshop supports the use of media campaigns where the above criteria are met and where local needs are adequately taken into account through consultation, research and evaluation.

No mass media program on drugs, either at a Commonwealth or State level, should be undertaken without some evidence of potential success, and in the case of Commonwealth campaigns consultation with all State Health Departments.

Wherever appropriate, a mass media program should have back-up support programs at a local level, built-in evaluation, adequate funding.

Liaison with the media should be pursued with a view to establishing guidelines for reporting substance-related matters.

All forms of advertising of tobacco should be banned, and a statutory code should be developed (replacing the present voluntary code) governing the advertising of alcohol. The interpretation of this should be vested in a body on which health, road safety and other consumer groups are adequately represented.

Sponsorship of sporting events based on the promotion of alcohol and tobacco should be phased out.

Properly planned and co-ordinated public education programs (via media and health promotion) should be implemented:

   to establish that the drug problem is everyone's problem
   to demystify community beliefs and attitudes
   to provide information and resources
   to assist communities to set agenda
   to foster an awareness of cultural differences
   to foster recognition that harm from legal drugs is greater than from illegal
   to create an understanding that drug problems are rarely caused solely by drug usage
   to raise community awareness that there is no 'quick fix'
   to increase public awareness of drug treatment programs which promote greater public acceptance of drug users and which counter their alienation from the community.

1. North Coast Healthy Lifestyle Program—New South Wales
See Section A, 'Community'.

2. Drink driving campaigns
Drink driving campaigns have been run both nationally and in the States in recent years. They have been sponsored by a number of organisations including the Federal Department of Transport, the State road safety and traffic authorities, the motorists' associations, the Australian Medical Association and the Australian Hoteliers' Association. The campaigns, which were particularly designed to cut down on holiday road tolls, have included informational and motivational components and made extensive use of TV and brochures.

3. Proposed new standards for advertising alcoholic liquor on television
In October 1984 the Australian Broadcasting Tribunal issued for comment proposed new standards. This action arose from considerable public concern that TV advertisements contained messages which associated alcoholic liquor with favourable lifestyles which would particularly appeal to young people, and

which were often being shown at hours when young people watched TV.

The proposed changes include restriction of timing and content and are at present being considered by all interested parties.

4. Movement against tobacco and alcohol sponsorship
While fully recognising the influence that tobacco and alcohol companies have on government, a number of concerned individuals and organisations have been attempting to raise public awareness and bring about change in sponsorship. Those most active in this ongoing lobbying have been the Health Authorities, Cancer Councils, the anti-smoking movement in general and particular individuals such as Senator Peter Baume. They have been supported in their efforts by stances taken by the Australian Institute of Sport, Actors Equity, the East Torrens District Cricket Club and various individual sports people who have refused such sponsorship.

5. Quit. For Life campaign
The Quit. For Life campaign was run in Sydney and in other parts of the country, under different names. Use of the media has been a major part of the campaign including dramatic (and controversial) TV advertisements.

The campaign aims both to discourage people, especially children, from starting to smoke and to help people who wish to give it up. It emphasises the importance of understanding the facts about smoking and what factors influence an individual's choice to use and abuse drugs.

Contact: Pallister House, Health, Media and Information Centre, North Sydney
Ph. (02) 4394288

G. Research

DA:NA recommendations
A national centre or institute of drug studies should be established with the following functions:
(a) to develop, evaluate and utilise data systems on drugs
(b) to evaluate social policy

(c) to initiate basic and applied research into drugs and the treatment of dependence
(d) to develop model cross-disciplinary education, training and treatment programs
(e) to promote exchange of ideas between professions and communities in Australia
(f) to provide a model of support and co-ordination of community drug programs developed by communities
(g) to provide a consultancy service—e.g. promote a public climate of co-operation between governments, media and the community.

The national centre should include the full range of relevant disciplines and the directorship should be drawn from any appropriate discipline. The centre should be adequately funded to enable it to achieve world standing.

A national institute should record all results of evaluation of treatment, educational and preventive programs.

1. Australian Institute of Alcohol and Drug Studies
Recently a proposal has been put forward to the government by Alcohol and Drug Foundation, Australia for a national institute which would have responsibility for establishing a national database for research, educational and policy purposes. It would oversee and co-ordinate research and become a centre of expertise and training.

2. National Health and Medical Research Council (NH&MRC)
NH&MRC has increased the amount of funds available for drug and alcohol research in recent years. It presently funds projects which include studies into the biochemistry of drug use, the psychiatric aspects of alcoholism, blood pressure, nutrition, smoking and treatment methods. It also funds the NH&MRC Road Accident Research Unit at Adelaide University.

3. University of New South Wales
Projects include studies into physician substance abuse, and an approach to smoking control and patterns of use of Benzodiazepines in Sydney.

4. Australian Associated Brewers
On the advice of its Medical Research Advisory Committee, a number of grants have been made in the past for studies into the

physiological, psychological and epidemiological aspects of alcohol consumption and the understanding and control of factors which modify the risk of alcohol- related medical problems.

5. Commonwealth Department of Health

Among the Health Services Research and Development Grants announced in August 1984 was one to review the Latrobe Valley Community Smoking Control Project, which has been designed to reduce over five years the incidence of smoking among adolescents in the Valley.

The Department of Health also collates research information from other sources and produces summaries, such as *Alcohol in Australia: a summary of related statistics*.

6. State governments

State governments also fund research, such as the New South Wales studies on drug use in pregnancy, cirrhosis of the liver in women, and effects of cannabis on drivers.

7. New South Wales Bureau of Crime Statistics and Research and Australian Institute of Criminology

Both of these agencies are involved in drug use research of various kinds, for instance on the sentencing of drug offenders in New South Wales and models for the custody of mentally disordered offenders.

8. Australian Medical Society on Alcohol and Drug Related Problems (AMSAD)

See Section C, 'Skills training: professionals and community'.

AMSAD, although it does not fund research, provides an Australian vehicle for the publication and exchange of research findings. It does this by holding annual conferences and by publishing the *Australian alcohol/drug review*.

H. Law

DA:NA recommendations

Such profits and assets of individuals and corporations as are accumulated through illicit drug trading should be confiscated legally, and should be applied in such proportion as is deemed appropriate by government for use in drug management programs.

We recommend, for drug users, the option of diversion from the legal system to treatment when appropriate facilities are available and acceptable to the individual. Where adequate facilities do not exist they should be made available.

Licensing restrictions are an important form of control in alcohol sales and need close evaluation and should be regularly reviewed and related to community needs and health considerations.

The illicit drug trade can generate corruption in every area of society. Recognising that this problem must be tackled at all levels, one obvious need is to ensure that direct law enforcement authorities each have fully empowered, adequately staffed internal investigatory bodies, with proper pursuit of convictions through the courts.

Special prescription forms for doctors to supply dangerous drugs (colour coded, serial numbered) should be introduced nationally.

Research into the relationships between drug abuse and crime must be supported and developed through the appropriate national and State research agencies.

Amongst the means available to influence the consumption of alcohol and tobacco, the following are recommended for implementation:

(a) The introduction of differential taxation reflecting the alcohol content of beverages and the tar content of cigarettes.

(b) An increase in real terms of the price of alcoholic beverages and tobacco and the price of alcoholic beverages and tobacco to be regularly reviewed in line with increased in the CPI so that their price, relative to disposable income, remains constant.

(c) The introduction of random breath testing in all States and Territories and the standardisation of the permissible blood alcohol level at 0.05.

(d) The review and revision of all crimes and penalties relating to alcohol and tobacco sale and use, with a view to ascertaining and improving their efficacy in reducing the harm associated with these drugs.

(e) Whilst the advertising of alcohol and tobacco remains, interpretation of the present voluntary codes is to be vested in bodies on which health and other consumer interests are adequately represented.

Some examples of State authorities working towards these principles are given.

1. The Drug and Alcohol Court Assessment Program (DACAP) —Sydney

This program, begun in 1980, goes some of the way to providing a comprehensive and rational approach to diversion and treatment of drug offenders which at present does not exist.

It provides a diversion by the legal system of a drug user to a health care system at the pre-sentence stage, so that the offender is offered intervention services but is still subject to the due process of law.

The diversion system involves linking a network of services which includes legal, correctional, health and voluntary organisations in a particular way. It works with street drug users through some city courts, e.g. Petty Sessions. The offender is put through a diagnostic process to assess special treatment needs and can be re-evaluated if the treatment is unsuccessful.

Contact: Drug and Alcohol Court Assessment Program,
Haymarket, Sydney
Ph. (02) 2176165

2. Smoking bans

The Victorian Government has recently banned smoking on public transport and related property throughout the State.

3. Blood alcohol levels

The New South Wales Transport Minister has recently proposed that the blood alcohol level for provisional drivers be set at zero and that that for supervising drivers should be under 0.05.

4. Self-regulation by advertisers

A Code of Advertising Ethics has been written by a number of committees and councils and was produced in booklet form by the Australian Advertising Industry Council in 1979 as a guide for both advertisers and agents in all States. Together they share the common objective of preventing the appearance of misleading or offensive advertising.

Through this industry self-regulation process, the advertising and media industry groups regulate the advertising activities of their members. Many operate under the umbrella of the Media Council of Australia and the Advertising Standards Council which is responsible for adjudicating complaints that particular advertisements breach the rules of industry self-regulation. The process is currently under review by many drug and alcohol authorities throughout Australia who are concerned at the lack of enforcement, and in some cases violation, of the code.

Contact: Australian Advertising Industry Council
Ph. (02) 9222300

5. Penalties for under age drinking

A South Australian Liquor Licensing Act of May 1985 significantly increased penalties for under age drinking and licensees were given greater powers to exclude young people from their premises. Under age drinkers can be removed from premises for failing to state their true age and will have to show proof of age.

It is also proposed that there be tougher penalties and increased powers for people operating dances and other forms of entertainment which young people are likely to attend.

The Act has proposed increased penalties up to $5000 for young people who consume alcohol on licensed premises.

6. Identity cards

The Queensland Minister for Justice has proposed that identity cards be instituted which can be presented by teenagers if challenged about their age in drinking places. They may be distributed through the State Electoral Office.

Major drug information agencies in Australia

National	Alcohol and Drug Foundation, Australia (ADFA) Ph. (062) 496888
Australian Capital Territory	Alcohol and Drug Service ACT Health Authority Ph. (062) 454111
New South Wales	Drug and Alcohol Authority Ph. (02) 2176163

Northern Territory	Drug and Alcohol Bureau Ph. (089) 802982
Queensland	Alcohol and Drug Dependence Service Ph. (07) 2296566
South Australia	Drug and Alcohol Services Council Ph. (08) 2743333
Tasmania	Alcohol and Drug Dependency Board Ph. (002) 306500
Victoria	Alcohol, Drug and Forensic Branch Health Commission of Victoria Ph. (03) 6167777
Western Australia	Alcohol and Drug Authority Ph. (09) 3212444

Adequacy of the national repertoire

The direct action reviewed here makes an impressive display. There can be no doubt that somewhere, sometime, all over Australia there are effective projects in the field of tackling drug abuse. We have no way of knowing how comprehensive our list is, although we do know how hard we tried to make it so. As it stands, however, we can make some comments on the national ability to service the National Campaign.

Education programs, that is formal programs for schools, are way out in front, and reflect the initiative of the National Drug Education Program. It is still disappointing to find so many of these programs in isolation from one another, or picked up in one State and not another. There is also a lack of the sort of comprehensive evaluation which would allow one group to build on another's work, or a new program to evolve from the old.

Community programs, although among the most challenging and interesting, are fewer than can meet the need indicated in the recommendations for the National Campaign. Media campaigns tend to be isolated from the communities they serve, with consequent risks of a backlash or evaporation of the messages. Notable exceptions are the Western Australian stop smoking program and the Pharmacists' Community Health Education Campaign in New South Wales, which have effectively focused on school and community.

Resources have been developed by the National Drug Education Program, local health centres and national groups such as Alcohol and Drug Foundation, Australia. There are undoubtedly excellent resources available (there ought to be, after so many major inquiries) but there are few central co-ordinating points or cross-referencing systems.

Skills training, the third naturally occurring category of existing action, appears excellent where it can be found. Available for teachers and in some central services, and usually applicable to all workers on drug abuse, it is not generally available to workers in the treatment services listed in Section E, 'Treatment and rehabilitation centres'. The establishment of AMSAD should help in this regard (see Section C, 'Skills training: professionals and community'). Even more serious is the absence of skills training in police colleges and preventive services. This is an area which came up repeatedly in the chapters on preventive strategies, and was also high on the list in recommendations for the National Drug Campaign.

In retrospect, it would appear that Australia has a better national repertoire of drug abuse prevention programs than it perhaps deserves, especially in the light of lack of action on Royal Commission recommendations in the past. However, there are serious gaps in evaluation, co-ordination, and access to information about various types of action, and it is to be hoped that in a year from now a more comprehensive review including all the fresh action will be available, and that the overall pattern of action will be more comprehensive.

Thus, of the two features necessary for successful social change (according to Schein, that is), we have seen that there is in Australia not only the 'pull' of the consensus on appropriate action by Premiers and public, but also people on the ground who can supply the action.

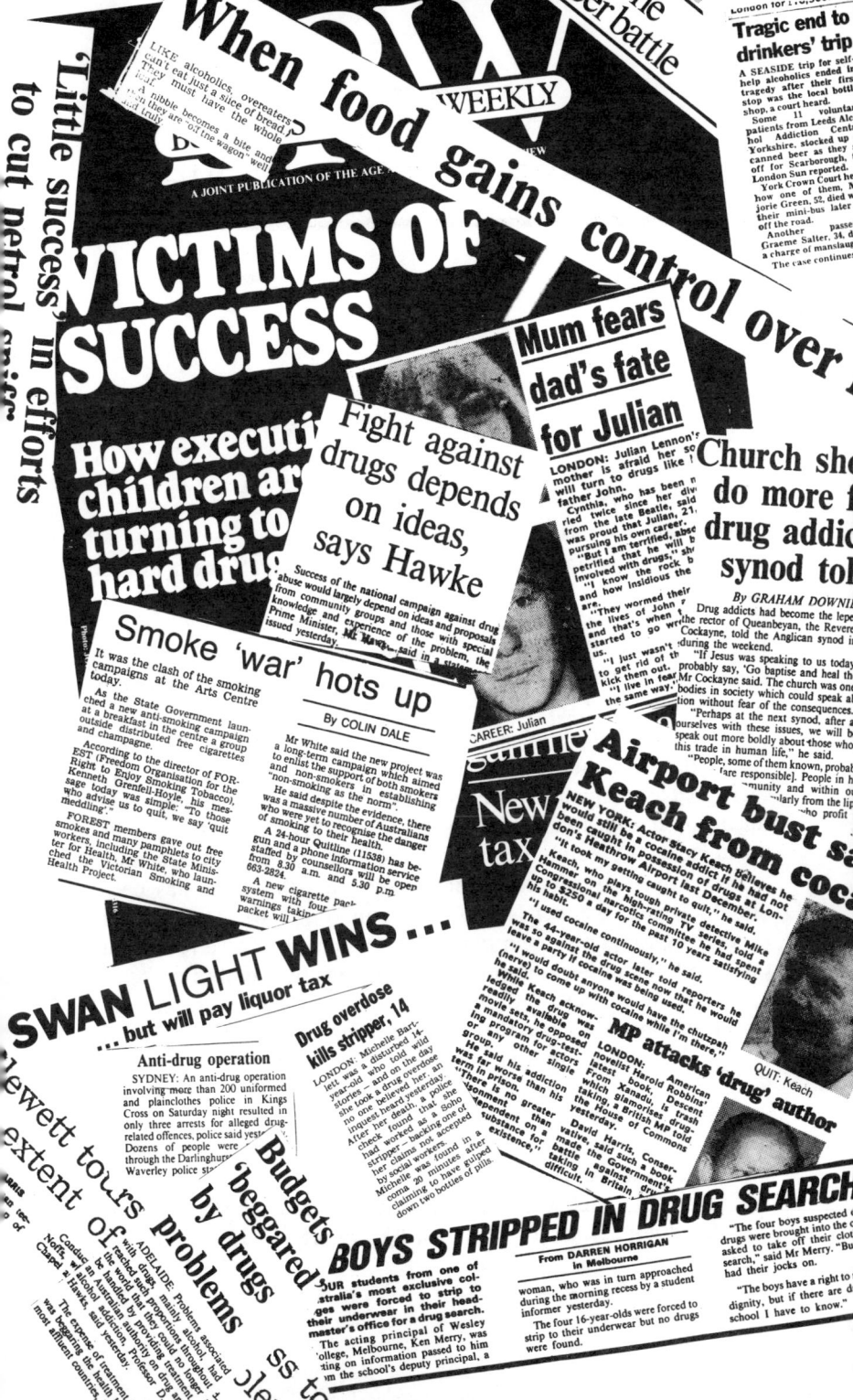

13
The Heart of the Matter

The status quo

Omens and portents

Number 13 as our last chapter has an ominous ring. Some buildings have no thirteenth floor, and some theatres no thirteenth seat, an idea that seems to have lingered past its time. Who does not know that the number thirteen is unlucky, and who now knows why that should be so? We can be sure that to have survived as a modern taboo it must still serve some human purpose.

The very word 'drug' seems to be as strongly linked to a taboo association as is number thirteen, and with as little (or as much) logic. It is synonymous with evil, corruption, physical decay and illicit power and, like all taboos, repels further examination of its meaning, so the clouds of suspicion are never dispelled. But neither is preventive action taken. And that is what this book has been about. Unless we can fight free from our own taboos, not necessarily to ignore them but to understand them, we remain at the mercy of, rather than in control of, our own daily fix.

At the beginning of Chapter 2 we played a game of tic-tac-totem, in which we learnt that the same drug can be both totem and taboo. This is not unusual; it is part of the rules of the game. A totem draws its power from two directions. First, from its ability to represent, in one sight or sound, our ethical, social and aesthetic rules as a coherent whole; so that whole becomes so powerful that who would dare question, even when the evidence of one's own eyes refutes it. Teachers in our infants classes have long known that they could not afford to see, much less report, the bruises on the bodies of 3 and 4-year-olds in their care. Until the last few years, the taboo which prevented the reporting of child abuse was the opposite and reinforcing side of the coin to motherhood, a totem which represented the absolute ethical goal of total devotion to another, the social rule that no one else had a right to an opinion on a child's welfare, and the aesthetic certainty that 'a child's place is with its mother'. For most of us our individual experience, miraculously, reinforced the totem, and so it continued unquestioned. It has only been after some of the elements of the totem have been called into question (women have claimed rights to other than total devotion to their children; men have asked to be included in those social and aesthetic rules regarding child care) that those whose experience does not fit with the totem have been able to be heard. It is less than five years since the first anonymous phone-in in Australia brought to public recognition the vulnerability of all mothers to abusing their children.

Taboos and totems
If it seems that the previous paragraph has not been related to the topic of drugs, then consider the following case. In the last year, a teacher from a middle class high school with three thousand pupils has come to one of the authors and said, I have the names of every heroin pusher in my school and there are thirteen of them. How did you get it, we said, and what will you do with it? She had been given the list by a student who admired and trusted her and who, far gone in addiction, was going to run away from home and school to a 'new' environment, to try to break free. Her family had no idea of her addiction. There is no need to dwell on her chances of success. The inner cities have many such refugees.

And what was the schoolteacher going to do with that knowledge and that list? Forget it, and burn it.

Before you judge harshly, as indeed I did at the time, consider the power of the taboo. Experience tells that teacher, a particularly open and responsive educator, that the parents would consider their child slandered if the teacher went to them, and it is against normal school behavioural rules for her to do so in the first place. The list of suppliers? Who would, or could, act? The evidence is not there; the students would protect each other; the staff do not want 'trouble'; the principal will not admit that there is heroin in 'his' school, any more than the parents can admit to themselves that 'their' daughter is a user. Police can only arrest; they cannot prevent or treat. *Go ask Alice* is a brilliant (and anonymous) book about such a dilemma. I was forced to concede, in this instance, that the teacher was absolutely correct. Her role as a confidante and her ability to help individuals was unique in her school, and the taboo was more effective than any law—than *the* law—in preventing remedial action. Before distancing ourselves from an illicit drug problem in an unknown school, try translating the whole issue to the alcoholic 14-year-olds, and the children of alcoholic parents in your own local high school. Both of these exist, you may be sure, at a rate of about one in ten. That figure is drawn from estimates, and from teacher observation; since the existence of child alcoholism is taboo, the figures cannot be verified, and so we do not have to believe them.

Another and related taboo is the link between parental modelling and child addiction. In nicotine consumption, we are able to establish that the greatest single predictable factor in whether a girl will smoke is whether her mother smokes. We can establish that because it has been permissible to ask, in school surveys, whether a parent smokes. Imagine the results if school children were asked how much alcohol does your mother, father drink each day, each week?

Yet we need this knowledge desperately. Workers in many treatment agencies are convinced that every client they see is an echo of a drug-abusing parent; only the drug being abused is different. From the inquiries by Baume and others, there is enough evidence on alcohol use among children of alcoholics to trace that direct link, even to the point that genetic transmission of alcoholism has been hypothesised. The links between alcohol as a drug of abuse in one generation, followed by cannabis and heroin in the next, cannot be established because of the illicit nature of the drug use; and not because there is a lack of evidence supporting the proposition.

The taboo here is doubly reinforced. Not only are questions about the use of illicit drugs, by definition, unaskable; the line between licit and illicit is a safety belt for the whole society, and must be kept sharp and clear. We must know which is which, they say, or how can we keep our totems and taboos? If the illegal drug of one era is the favoured drug of the next, as Table 4 in Chapter 2 would indicate, are we bound to a wheel? Unquestioned totems and taboos certainly maintain that wheel. Is the sniffing of solvents, emerging among young children and some disadvantaged groups, the next addiction? The French have a saying, the more things change, the more they stay the same. Perhaps the only choice we have is to decide the manner in which totems will be kept, and reduce the number of taboos we are prepared to observe.

Here and now
We can do no more here than to point out the present members of our society at risk from their daily fixes, and link these to the more obvious social taboos. What happens next lies in the future, but a future in which there appears to be a considerable national will to stop the turning wheel.

A summary of the known patterns of drug use and abuse gives us this quick snapshot.

Statistics on use of legal drugs (alcohol, nicotine, analgesics and tranquillisers) suggest that their use is increasing among young females and the elderly, staying level among young males and the middle-aged (40-50 years) of both sexes, with a decrease in nicotine use among adults between 35 and 45 years, and bulges in the use of alcohol for both sexes in the early twenties and fifties. Alcohol-related car driver deaths are decreasing, but those of pedestrians and at high speed are increasing. In spite of a decrease in Australian road deaths, it remains true that one in ten of Australian male youths will be permanently damaged by a road accident, half of which are alcohol related.

The use of legal drugs in pregnancy has been curtailed, but the overuse of analgesics by (mostly) women still gives us the highest rate of kidney disease in the world; and the rate of consumption of alcohol puts us among the highest users in the western world, as does the consumption of tranquillisers. Before we touch on the matter of illegal drugs, we have to concede that we are a nation of drug users.

The use of illegal drugs has to be estimated from straws in the wind. Increase in amounts seized by police may simply reflect increased efficiency; an increase in prosecutions and gaol sentences may reflect increased intolerance of the practices concerned. Nevertheless, it seems certain that there was an extremely rapid increase in both supply and use of heroin in Australia in the late 1970s: an increase which had been clearly predicted by Customs officials and workers in the drug field, both here and overseas. Even though the increase may be as great as tenfold, about three per cent of 16 to 30-year-olds are estimated as users of heroin today. About half of those will return to society, free of their habit, while the rest will deteriorate and be permanently incapacitated or die. Cocaine is following the same track, with the differences of greater crime (it is much more expensive than heroin) and less physiological damage to the user, at least in the short term.

Can we connect this overview with our present social taboos? It isn't very difficult, and the advertising agents have been doing it for decades. Let us take the drugs discussed above in turn.

Alcohol with its religious symbolism, its place in social celebrations, and its role in release from alienating work roles, is a totem which one cannot imagine replaced. A taboo is placed on discussion of the drinking of alcohol by women, who have less physiological capacity to absorb the drug, and a potential to damage the next generation, as foetus and dependent child. The competing totem of social equality for women reinforces this taboo. For men, the totem of the manly qualities of strength and endurance cannot be questioned by setting limits to alcohol capacity, particularly where the society is resting on the use of alcohol to keep workers in unpalatable jobs, or the unemployed less discontented with their lot. Here we have one example of the preservation of the symbolism of a totem with a change in the actual physical form. Low alcohol beers, runaway bestsellers in spite of all market prediction, allow the preservation of the symbolic behaviours (long hours of drinking with mates, relaxed and sometimes antisocial behaviours, women drinking at the same rates as men), at no cost to the market forces, or to the individual's physiological fitness. There would seem to be considerable scope for raising the acceptability of small quantities of alcohol (supported by studies of its lowering risk of heart disease, presumably as a release for stress), and maintaining the totem, with its socially desirable aspects. This optimistic note must be tempered by reporting the distinct trend of the mid-teen drinkers of alcohol to moving to spirits and hard liquor. Those soft-drink bottles so innocently brought to your child's first grown-up party—smell them. The colour can mask rum, gin or whisky.

The epidemic in the 1970s of Valium prescription for women has abated—or has it? Its use coincided with the taboo against questioning that women in Australia were the happiest of mortals, secure in their husband's protection and the well-deserved rewards of a lifelong devotion to their children. The statistics of the time show a 50 per cent increase in divorce rates (and remarriage rates), a steadying of reproduction rates to the 2.3 children of today, and the start of the custom of 18-year-olds living independently of their families (thus less than one-half of a mother's working life is actually devoted to caring for her children). Over half married women were in the workforce, including one-third of those with small children. No wonder the conflict between ideal and reality caused depression and stress—and several authors, including Dorothy Broom, have described the response meted out to women who turned to another of our social totems for help. Women and men presenting with exactly the same symptoms of occupational stress were given quite different medical treatments. While the women were supplied tranquillisers, men were advised to change their jobs, use sports and relaxation, or alter their working conditions. Taboos on discussing the social realities had brought another totem into play: medication, the supply of the (legitimately) wonder drugs of our age. There is a chemical solution to everything; so there must be a chemical solution to this epidemic of female unhappiness. The totem's use outlasted the first-hand knowledge of the long-term effects of such tranquillisers (addiction and mental disorientation) by over a decade. Although the use of the traditional tranquillisers has now dropped sharply, as the tables compiled for the Drug Summit show, they have been replaced by others; the totem triumphs, the taboo holds.

Illegal and illicit drugs (and they are not the same thing), although taboo in themselves, are, as we have already observed, totems to the sub-culture of their users. It is, on the other hand, taboo to acknowledge that once a heroin user not always a heroin user (in fact, the rate of physical addiction is quite slow, taking weeks of use), that withdrawal, under proper medical supervision, can be relatively painless (it must be upheld as a dreadful punishment for use), that use is not confined to the criminal element (your own child, as we have indicated, can almost certainly get it from school, and you yourself from several of the downtown bars). If you can find the money to pay for heroin, have the self-control to limit your use, and can find an unadulterated source of supply (all pretty difficult, not to say impossible), you could use heroin for a lifetime, as is perfectly well known to the users, and to the treatment agencies. But since it is socially more acceptable to control by totem and taboo than by reason, we cling to the taboo.

This is where we are, in terms of drug use, as a nation, now. In terms of prevention of abuse, where are we going?

Quo vadis?

The directions in which the main avenues of response to drug abuse are going are encouraging, as we have discussed extensively in Part 2. Workers in the fields of control, treatment, education and social change are all at present reconsidering their various positions and there are indications, encouraged by the recommendations of the recent range of drug workshops, that the various professional groups acknowledge the need to work together on the issues. Parallel, and important, social trends are the recognition that control and treatment are not ends in themselves, but links in a chain of prevention and rehabilitation; that education is not a soft option in which the mere knowledge of the issues is sufficient to solve the problems; and that we are living in a time of acute social change, a fact which we ignore at our peril.

All of these phenomena have been recognised in the funding for the National Drug Campaign, and we have suggested a pentagon method of evaluation which could monitor the extent to which they are actually taken into account in subsequent professional programs. It is worth reviewing the various frameworks we have been offering, to see how one could expect them to be used in the future.

Table 1 provided an overview of recommendations for drug policy, strategy and action over the last fifteen years. This is a benchmark against which action and change can be reassessed in years to come; even if, as a rather world weary Earle Hackett tells us in the Postscript that follows, there is really very little of either. Figure 1 presents a policy-to-action wheel, which in our discussion, and in most current social expectation, is assumed to turn anti-clockwise. That is, we assume that we must thoroughly study the status quo in our society, and use the currently acceptable strategies, in order to apply policies for successful action. We can now suggest, in the light of our later discussion of social change, that perhaps it is a time for turning the wheel clockwise. If a policy is to put pressure on totems, and question taboos, then the action needed may be to find new strategies, and to alter the social context itself. At first hearing, an impossibly difficult task, until one considers Margaret Mead's rational analysis of a fast-changing society with its need to learn from its own young, who haven't learnt all the mistakes (yet); and the sensitive and thoughtful considerations of community development which are emerging in the literature.

Australia has seen a transmutation from a British-based, nineteenth century social system to a rich mix in which one in three children have a non English-speaking grandparent; in which wine drinking has changed from dingy, secluded bars to every dinner table; in which the foods available have changed from plain roast or boiled to an elaborate and exciting range, a joy to dietary, social and aesthetic senses; and in which we are now locked in a controversy on whether we can afford to continue the transmutation, or whether it is time to cement our population as it stands now. Social change and social dissent are always with us, but particularly so now. Drug issues are not separate from the other issues, but they are often used to distract attention from them.

In Tables 2 and 7, we tried to provide a framework whereby the drug issues of the day could be addressed in relation to their social setting, but not be used as scapegoats, or witch hunts, both popular social mechanisms for avoiding rational discussion. Having drawn on the seminal work of Helen Nowlis, we have related the most highly developed strategies for prevention of drug abuse to the aspects of evidence each type of strategist needs to consider. In doing this, we also provided a common framework, so that a physician, who might rely heavily on empirical evidence of physical effects, could draw on the knowledge of social rules held by lawyers and the police, and the knowledge of how individuals think and feel, developed by the educators.

This integration of the various professional efforts is also encouraged by a general trend in professional education to involve the client more in the service, whether it is the prisoner in their own rehabilitation, the patient in taking responsibility for their own health, the teacher in involving students in the preparation of the curriculum, or the community worker who develops self-help groups among those in need. All these trends, although they have not been so labelled, are variants of Mead's prefigurative learning. The elders, the wise, the trained professionals in a time of social change must listen to the community-at-large; expert knowledge must be continually re-evaluated to see if it is still effective. Evaluated not discarded, one notes; the baby out with the bathwater syndrome is as wasteful of generations of social learning as is the fixed-vision dinosauric view.

All these trends towards diversity and co-ordination of services, of responsiveness rather than fence sitting, lead not to a firm path but to an uncertain future full of risk taking, ambiguity and paradoxes. We have invented a rather more sophisticated game than tic-tac-toe for workers with drug issues; a game which reflects the interplay between totems and taboos, the incongruities between different choices of treatment, and the sheer element of chance. Figure 12 represents our summing up of the future to be expected in reducing drug abuse—a continuing game of Snakes and Ladders.

The rules of the game

When it comes to action, the various issues surrounding a drug problem must be resolved, for good or ill. The very decision to act names the game. A large number of unpredictable factors then come into play. The initial intervention forces one or other type of solution on the issue; that solution is then carried this way and that by what are sometimes called market forces, and sometimes called chance; so the game is not unlike Snakes and Ladders. Sometimes the result is positive and one moves forward, with reduced drug use, and rehabilitated abusers. Sometimes a shipment of adulterated heroin finally destroys the health of a group of youngsters whom a therapist has just persuaded to accept detoxification; sometimes a family travels across Australia, having found a program which they believe is suitable for their drug-addicted child, only to have the program collapse for want of funds. Yet another family is happily consolidating its position with a parent who has joined Alcoholics Anonymous, when the parent loses his or her job, and the pressures become too great for sobriety to last.

The game is a series of interactions between the problem-solving levels of policy, strategy, action and social context (expanded in Chapter 1); between the avenues of control, treatment, education

THE HEART OF THE MATTER 265

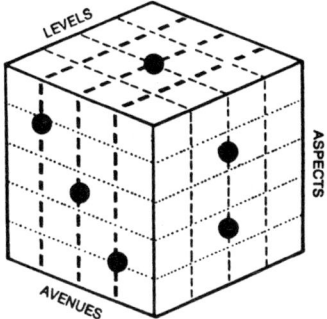

Figure 11   A loaded dice?

To play

1. Take a dice. Each *plane* represents a move:

    if you throw a six or a one, move one
    if you throw a five or a two, move two
    if you throw a four or a three, move three.

2. Each player takes it in turn to roll the dice, and move the number indicated. If you are in square 3 and throw a three, go to square 6. Follow the instructions on the square you land in; for example, *back one space* or *miss two turns*. Each square represents an aspect of the problem appropriate to that particular intersection of level and avenue: thus one particular control-policy is tough penalties for cannabis use (square 5), one treatment-strategy is methadone (10), and so on.

3. A number of squares have the phrase *next go*: accompanied by three options. These represent three possible outcomes of the scenario contained in that square. On your next turn, throw the dice and follow the outcome indicated. For example, if you land in square 14, on your next go if you throw a one or two take the snake to square 6, and if you throw a three go to *finish*.

4. If the outcome is *stay put,* then don't do anything. The next time it is your turn, you can go forward according to the throw of the dice. That is, if you *stay put* on square 5, a three next turn will move you on to square 8.

5. On square 16, you must throw a one to move forward to the *finish*. Social change activism can be successful, unsuccessful, or its effects can be postponed. It cannot merely be circumvented.

266 OUR DAILY FIX

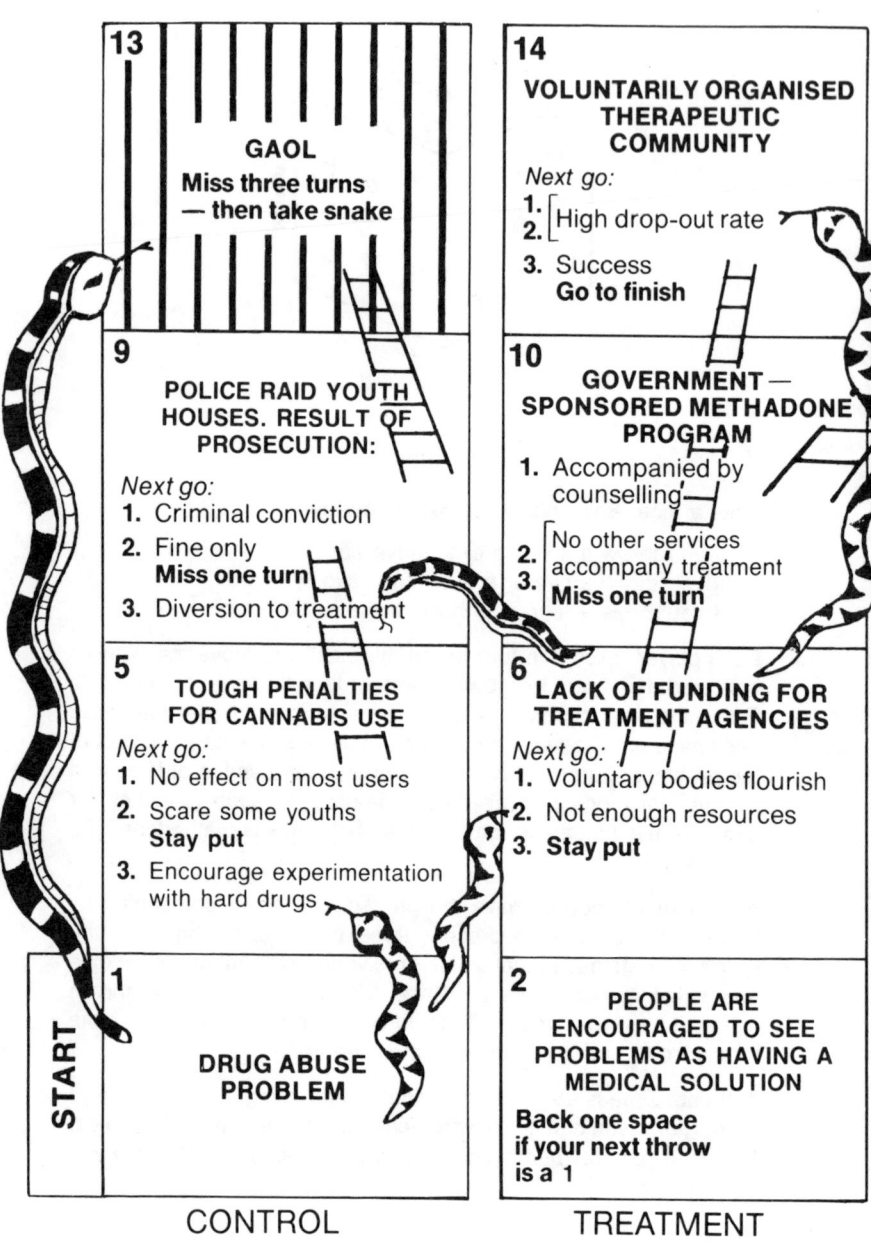

Figure 12 Snakes and ladders

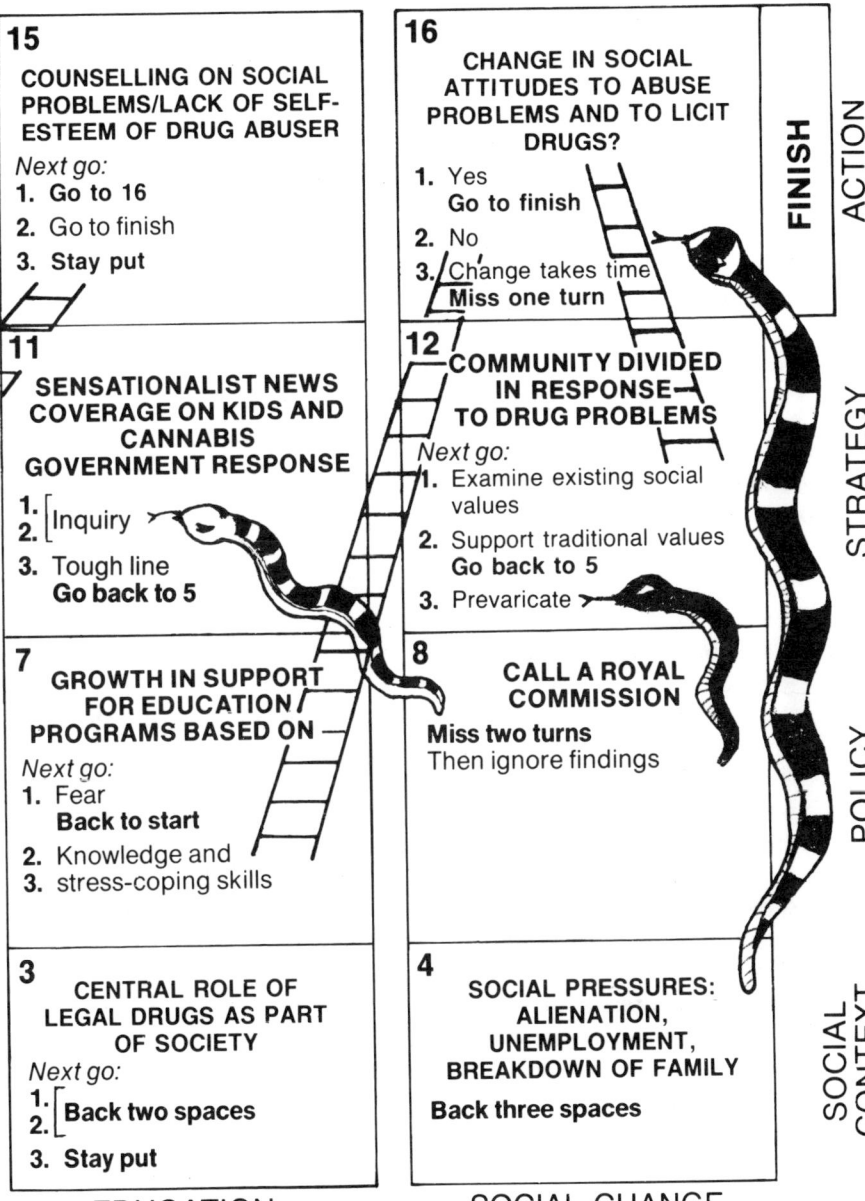

and social change as the means of prevention (clarified in Chapter 3); and between the physical, ethical, aesthetic, and social aspects of the issues involved (defined in Chapter 5); the three planes of a dice which many believe to be loaded representing the three dimensions which must be considered to gain a proper perspective. Whether loaded or not, the game in Figure 12 is played with that dice and is played for real. The rules are the same as for any game of chance, and you win if you have balanced use and abuse of a drug so that the balance will hold. In this book we have been providing a detailed description of the way in which the dice is constructed, which should help in discovering whether it throws true. Whether the game is crooked or not depends upon where and with whom you are playing.

Q.E.D.

Did we set out to prove anything? A claim to prove anything at all in the field of drug abuse would be presumptuous indeed. But we must admit to an attempt to prove several propositions; not in the sense of establishing beyond doubt, but in the slightly older and more liberal sense of putting to the test. To prove a metal is to put it under severe conditions to see if it will stand up to the strain. In this book we have offered the thesis that there is no Australian unaffected by their own or others' use of drugs, and no one of us untouched by the effects of abuse. We then set out to prove (in the sense of test) the propositions; first, that it is possible to understand the drug use of people or communities alien to us, or even of ourselves, which is far more difficult. Second, we have tried to show the connections and relationships between use and abuse of chemical agents, so that usual social divisions between legal and illegal, licit and illicit, dependence and choice, addiction and freedom, oppressor and victim, professional and client can be reconsidered, and so re-evaluated. We have presented a fivefold form of evaluation which may be able to stand up to the difficult task of re-examining the very totems and taboos by which we structure our thinking. We have incorporated the five aspects of evidence on drug issues, by reviewing the evidence on physical effects of drugs and the extent of their use; the ethical goals we are likely to find in our society, and their influence on policy and politicians; the social rules which encompass our behaviour in taking drugs; the aesthetic choices which we may find difficult to explain, but which are powerful influences for all that; and finally we have surveyed the range of individual positions on drug issues as reflected in the spate of workshops and public statements across the country at the start of the National Campaign Against Drug Abuse. We have listed the range of services, resources, programs and projects available to those prepared to take on the task of reducing abuse.

We have not felt obliged to explain either the criminality or the economics of drug use and abuse. We have had both a lawyer and an economist in our team, and we take those issues seriously. We believe, however, that the first of these is a social effect, and the second a social tool, each subject to the same tools of analysis as we have employed here. Application of those tools to criminal subcultures, or the specialist field of supply-side economics, is the stuff of two further books, but not the one we have written here. This book took its shape from a commitment by the authors to brief a well-informed cross-section of the Australian community on the state-of-the-art in prevention of drug abuse, and the subsequent commitment of that group to finding realistic solutions to the problems involved.

Thus, we have kept to our main theme, our daily fix, and concentrated on those aspects of the drug problem that we can all do something about. Not simplistically, as in discouraging all drug use, but by discovering how to use drugs well. Not by being narrowly chauvinist, but considering all available solutions without succumbing to the very real possibility of other cultures, other eras, and other interests imposing their fixes on us. Not by being too idealistic, and waiting for a perfect world, but by looking to the essential structures of our society, the political lobbies, the professional help, the community solidarity, the family loyalties, and the personal power which is our strongest resource in the ups and downs of daily life. And that is the heart of the matter.

Postscript

Attending the Drug Workshop in Canberra gave me a feeling of *déjà vu*, for nine years ago I was a member of the Sackville Royal Commission. That had involved me for almost two years in hearing all the reiterated positions regarding drugs, accompanied by the shrill chorus kept up by the media. I remember that at that time I had written privately to a very experienced medical acquaintance who had spent his whole professional career advising the Home Office in London on the Drug Problem. I asked him to distil all his experience for me. He replied promptly. What the Drug Problem needs, he said wearily, is a good dose of boredom.

How to provide that I don't know. Perhaps a century of excited discussion by everybody, with full media responses, would do the trick. Then the Drug Problem might defuse into cool pharmacology and bare social statistics.

A day or so thinking about it is not enough even for 'experts', and certainly not enough for parliamentary debating chambers to reach any but the old kneejerk conclusions, as all western democracies have discovered.

For the Drug Problem is a mislabelled portmanteau, like the Abortion Question. Open the portmanteau and you find unconscious human needs to discuss things not on the label.

The Abortion Question is said publicly by zealots to be about murder but it turns out 'really' to be about unresolved attitudes to sexual freedom for young women.

The Drug Problem is said publicly by zealots to be about addiction and police work, but it turns out 'really' to be about unresolved attitudes to neurochemical by-passing of the human motivation to work, and about the fear that your children will become changelings.

Deeply felt approval/disapproval judgments surge up around what we (and others) believe we ought to be doing. Right versus wrong. Good versus evil. Anger. Envy. Guilt.

Until familiarity (or boredom as my medical friend called it) defuses these feelings in most people (that is not only in the breasts of experts but in those of the electorate) there will be no cool, rational resolving of the Drug Problem.

In the Workshop, our Australian dislike of philosophical or moral analysis was strong. The secular syndicates muttered throughout their first day like gangs of chained felons. Nobody was able to think out any general policy position until a flintlock was put to the heads of the Policy Syndicate. Then the quick wording they belatedly produced was strangely reminiscent of Sackville (which I happened to know was very reminiscent of Le Dain). Had we been in clear-thinking France there would have been entire structuralist, theist, existentialist, Marxist and anarchist policies offered for us workshoppers to choose from. In the Canberra Workshop, we largely ignored even the proffered belated policy guidelines and straightaway we chose minutiae. Thus we did not have to look at the difficult wood; we preferred to see easy trees.

The outcome, although a monument of small prejudices and compromises, was a lot of trees that probably added up to much the same sort of wood that we would have got had we started the other way round and scratched, patched and adapted an original ideal social policy. Pragmatism, decency and ignorance, well-mixed, usually get as far as a philosopher king on Australia Day.

Many participants held on to Manichean attitudes. They saw different drugs as either good or evil. Few saw the various substances as chemical or pharmacological entities. Others classified them more or less as friends, companions, neighbours, strangers, enemies or criminals.

Sackville in 1978 had recommended partial legalisation of cannabis when the politicians felt the time was ripe. I had agreed then, partly because of two years thinking, partly on medical grounds, and partly because as a rational tax-paying citizen I was against comic operatics in which huge bold gendarmeries pursued little boys whose offence was they had handfuls of dried leaves; not to mention the black economies which this created; and the corruption.

But the politicians were unconvinced, as they have been in most parts of the world after surprisingly similar reports. However, at the time of Sackville, perhaps only 20 per cent of the electorate took that liberalising view. A plenary session of the Workshop, though, suggested that now in 1985 the soften-up-on-cannabis vote is more like 50 per cent. Still not enough. The bold gendarmes will still chase the little boys. Heigh ho.

More important (for cannabis is, in any long-term view, a trivial public health matter) there would in 1978 have been only about 10 per cent in favour of classifying tobacco and alcohol as real drugs of addiction. Now the Workshop showed a large majority in favour. A pointer for the politicians, poor things, as they struggle with the art of the possible.

Obviously cannabis is slowly moving towards a disapproved but tolerated position, which for it implies some relaxation of public attitudes. Tobacco and alcohol, on the other hand, are equally slowly being acknowledged as the real Australian Killers and so they are becoming less tolerated, which for them means a tightening of attitudes. But it is a slow business. Each social initiative such as a workshop certainly contributes its tiny socio-historical mite towards a rational attitude to drugs, and another towards the eventual achievement of that national creative boredom which my friend so accurately discerned was a prerequisite for solving the Drug Problem.

Earle Hackett, M.D.
Adelaide, March 1985

Notes For Further Reading

We have avoided detailed referencing within the chapters, in order to make reading easier. Details of the sources of our information and opinions can be found in the Bibliography. In these Notes we provide some basic and/or background reading for each chapter, so that those who wish to delve more deeply in any area may do so. The readings are also intended to supply teaching materials for those developing courses in the area.

Chapter 1   The world in our heads: totems and taboos

An excellent overview of different professional perspectives on drugs in the Australian context is provided by the proceedings of the 1st Pan-Pacific Conference on Drugs and Alcohol, edited by Drew et al., entitled *Man, drugs and society—current perspectives*. Helen Nowlis in *Drugs demystified* manages, in a few short pages, to clarify the role of drugs in our lives, and to give constructive suggestions for what to do before drug taking gets out of hand. Mary Douglas provides a brilliant analysis of the way in which what we eat, the parts of our bodies, and our family relationships provide the powerful symbols from which we construct our world, in *Purity and danger* and also in *Natural symbols*. From there it is a short step to understanding how the use of drugs, legal and illegal, both reinforces and threatens our established world. A sensitive and understanding account of the ways in which drugs are taken, and the effects that they have on the human mind, is given by Andrew Weil in *The natural mind*.

Chapter 2 The social context of drug use

A useful frame of reference for a social analysis of drugs is given by Krivanek in *Drug problems, people problems*. The sociocultural and historical perspective is also well documented in Edwards et al., *Drug use and misuse: cultural perspectives*. Valuable for both this and the following chapter on drug policy is the book edited by Edwards and Arif, *Drug problems in the sociocultural context: a basis for policies and programme planning*.

For the reader interested in developing a deeper understanding of the meanings of drugs in our own society, there is much interesting material, some examples of which are: Mugford's *Australian drinking patterns: a legacy for our children*; *Cannabis and culture* by Rubin; Gusfield's *The culture of public problems: drink-driving and the symbolic order*; Trice and Roman's *Spirits and demons at work: alcohol and other drugs on the job*; and Walker's *Under fire: a history of tobacco smoking in Australia*.

For those with a research orientation, there is an excellent issue of *Journal of drug issues* in Winter 1984, edited by Rachin, called 'The orientation of sociology toward alcohol and society'. Similarly, all the volumes of the series "Research advances in alcohol and drug problems" are of interest, but especially volume 5, edited by Kalant, *Alcohol and drug problems in women*. An interesting perspective can be found in *Drinking and alcoholism in Australia: a power relations theory*, by Sargent.

A classic Australian paper, perhaps ahead of its time when issued by the Australian Foundation on Alcoholism and Drug Dependence (now ADFA) in 1982, is *Social policies on drugs: alcohol, cannabis, heroin*.

For the most balanced view on 'types' of drug user and drug-using environments, see Chapters 10-12, 24 and 25 of the *Handbook on drug abuse* edited by Dupont et al. For a subjective understanding of what it is like to change one's consciousness through drugs, there is Castaneda's *The teachings of don Juan*.

Chapter 3 Drug policy, politics and values

A classic book which allows readers to develop their own ideas about the uses of policy is Titmuss's *Social policy*. Unfortunately there are few works in the area of drugs which discuss the broad principles of the issues involved. A Canadian inquiry chaired by Le

Dain, *Commission of inquiry into the non-medical use of drugs*, is a useful exception to this rule. A good source for considering the relationship between Australian values and drug taking is. Peter Baume's report *Drug problems in Australia: an intoxicated society?* Delivered as long ago as 1977, the issues raised there are still surprisingly fresh—and unresolved.

The role of the press in moulding fears and concerns and setting agenda for policy is discussed in Bell, *Headlining drugs* and Windschuttle, *Drugs and the press*, the last being produced for the Sackville Royal Commission. For those who would like to pursue the ideas of policy and values into the field of ethics, *A short history of ethics* by MacIntyre is an easy introduction to the topic.

The reading suggested for Chapter 2 is mostly relevant here. For a masterly overview of the politics of one drug issue, read Taylor's *Smoke ring: the politics of tobacco*.

Chapter 4   Effects and extent of drug use

The most comprehensive yet readable reference on the nature of drugs is *Drugs and drug abuse* by Cox et al. For a more general, and Australian, reference, the Centre for Education and Information on Drugs and Alcohol has recently produced *An Australian handbook on drug use*.

For statistics on drug use and abuse, there are regular bulletins produced by the Australian Bureau of Statistics. The most recent major sources are *Statistics on drug abuse in Australia*, put out in 1985 by the Commonwealth Department of Health, and from which most of the statistics in this book are drawn; and *Risk-factor prevalence study, no. 2—1983*, produced by the National Heart Foundation.

Chapter 5   Our heads in the world

The difficulties in moving from theory to practice, with the associated problem of rationally analysing what is in part a leap of faith, have been a theme of many writers. The relationship between theory and practice is so interwoven, and the difficulty of clarifying the nature of the strategy step in between is so considerable, that a word—praxis—has been coined for this nexus between the world in the head and the head in the world. For those whose main concern is with the nature of human action, there is the classic by

Habermas, *Knowledge and human interests*, which tackles the problem at a theoretical level. Building on Habermas's propositions, Anthony Giddens is somewhat more practical, and in *Central problems in social theory: action, structure and contradiction in social analysis* he links some of the outstanding theoretical insights of this era to the problems of the planner and decision maker.

The method of choosing a strategy which is proposed in this chapter, that is, combining all aspects of the evidence in a holistic view, is amplified by one of the authors, Valerie A. Brown, in two papers which apply this method to health care research ('From sickness to health: an altered focus for health-care research', in *Social science and medicine*) and illness prevention ('Towards an epidemiology of health': a basis for planning community health programs', in *Health policy)*.

Chapter 6   Control

All the recent Royal Commissions have spent a great deal of space dealing with questions of legal controls. On questions of international measures, and supply-side steps such as Customs, coastal surveillance, and so on, Williams's *Australian Royal Commission* is very comprehensive. But that work, as with many others, does not examine its premises or state its value judgments. Therefore in dealing with more value-laden issues such as the legalisation of marijuana or whether there should be a crime of possession, the most thoughtful and valuable Royal Commission is that chaired by Professor Sackville. The report is well worth reading.

The *Bulletin of narcotics* (1983) devoted volume 35, part 2 to the profits of trafficking and their recovery. More generally, Wardlaw's excellent book *Drug use and crime* examines the myth and reality of the relationship between drugs and crime.

There are many other good contributions to particular areas of debate, such as the discussion papers put out by the Sackville Royal Commission (for example, Goode on *Drugs and the law*), and the papers put out by the New South Wales Drug and Alcohol Authority (for example, by Williams on *The drug and alcohol court assessment program*). In the area of legal drugs, Moser's publication on *Prevention of alcohol-related problems* is clear and detailed; Braithwaite's *Corporate crime in the pharmaceutical industry* is thorough and hard-hitting. From the other side of the legal fence, we have Dobinson and Ward on *Drugs and crime: a survey of N.S.W. prison property offenders*.

Chapter 7   Treatment

For a thoroughgoing discussion of the different attitudes to treatment as the only possible answer and as an exploitative monopoly, Taylor's *Medicine out of control* is sometimes entertaining, sometimes polemic, but always interesting. An older and more sedate book on the same theme is the classic *Medical nemesis* by Illich. For a masterly analysis of Australia's health services as a whole and how they got to be the way they are, read Sax's *A strife of interests: politics and policies in Australian health services* (although there is very little about drugs per se).

Articles which provide information on treatment, and at the same time give a perspective on the treatment, treater, and client, are those by Henderson, 'Substance use/abuse conceptualisation, etiology and treatment' in *Journal of drug issues* and by Ricketts and Nanra on 'Analgesic abuse in perspective' in *Australian alcohol/drug review*. Specialist journals such as *Journal of contemporary drug problems*, *International journal of the addictions*, *Australian alcohol/drug review*, and *Advances in alcohol and substance abuse* are a constant source of the details of new approaches to treatment. The whole issue of volume 3, part 4 of the last-mentioned journal, edited by Kreek and Stimmel, is particularly valuable for its evaluation of treatments in use at the moment.

Books and papers are also constantly issued by the United States National Institute on Drug Abuse, and Alcohol and Drug Foundation, Australia. This last is a recent change of name, and so materials may more often be found under the old name Australian Foundation on Alcoholism and Drug Dependence, Canberra.

Chapter 8   Education

The tight links between education, health education and socially sensitive areas such as drugs are outlined in principle by Green et al. in *Health education planning: a diagnostic approach*. This book is a fund of ideas for program planning, design and evaluation. For more specific ideas, and for evaluation of others' failures and successes, there are the specialist journals, *Journal of drug education* and *Journal of drug and alcohol education*. There is also a wide range of health education journals, which regularly print articles on drug education and preventive mechanisms.

If you are teaching or working with adults, Knowles's text on the nature of adult learning would be invaluable, although it doesn't mention drugs. For Australian ideas and materials, see the *Drug education guidelines* of the National Working Party for the Drug Education Project, put out by the Curriculum Development Centre in Canberra; Roger's paper on 'Strategy for drug abuse prevention' in Wardlaw (1982); and Irwin's paper on *Education and the use of alcohol and drugs*. An international perspective can be found in the World Health Organization paper by Vuylsteek on *Health education: smoking, alcoholism, drugs*. Chapter 12 of this book contains an annotated overview of education programs in use in Australia at the time of DA:NA.

Chapter 9   Social change

Toffler's *Future shock* and Mead's *Culture and commitment: the new relationships between the generations in the 1970's* together give a practical profile to the effect of our era of rapid change on ourselves, our society, and our social customs. Both are positive orientations towards harnessing social change, and making the new an improvement on the old. For an analysis of social change with factors which encourage and inhibit, read Schon's *Beyond the stable state*.

While there is a considerable literature on prevention of drug use and abuse, as for instance the Schaps et al. series on *Balancing head and heart: sensible ideas for the prevention of drug and alcohol abuse* and the National Institute on Drug Abuse paper on *Preventing adolescent drug abuse: intervention strategies*, edited by Glynn et al., most of it refers, as the titles suggest, to individual strategies for individual problems. For prevention on a larger, more co-ordinated scale we need to go to the general community development literature. In Australia, one cannot do better than to read Scott's *Don't mourn for me—organise* and Deveson's *Australians at risk*, for ideas of the major part the ordinary citizen can play, and the extent of the daily pressures in Australian lives, respectively. To identify current pressures and current solutions, the best source is the various journals which review social issues: *Journal of social issues*, *Australian journal of social issues*, and *New society*, *New doctor* and even *New scientist*. The most useful of all, because of its professed aim to unite theory and practice, is *Australian society*.

For a battery of techniques by which to affect or effect social change in a socially responsible manner, there are the three volumes of Sharpe's *The politics of non-violent action*. For one particular technique, the search conference, which has been successfully used as a tool for many groups and many cultures to adopt to their fast-changing world, there is *Futures we're in* by Fred Emery et al.

Chapter 10   Changing the world

This chapter, like Chapters 1 and 5, provides a theoretical framework for the following section. Thus the reading for this chapter is more appropriately related to evaluation of what went before, in order to make sound judgments in the future, than directly to drug issues. Classic works on evaluation include Parlett and Hamilton's *Evaluation as illumination*, writings by Scriven on goal-free evaluation and Stake on responsive evaluation, and Stufflebeam's *Educational evaluation and decision-making*.

For the particular evaluation method developed in this section, the background papers are those of Brown, listed in the reading for Chapter 5; a further paper, 'Five-dimensional evaluation', is in preparation. For the basis of the analysis of evidence which provides the theoretical framework of the five-dimensional evaluation, see three critiques of scientific method: Popper's *Objective knowledge*, Polanyi's *Personal knowledge*, and Toulmin's *Human understanding*. For a more digestible and even enjoyable overview of the synthesis of the subjective and objective in human reasoning there is Pirsig's *Zen and the art of motorcycle maintenance*.

Chapter 11   A national campaign against drug abuse

Since there has not been a precedent for this brave attempt to conduct a national campaign against drug abuse, we can only document the birth of this one, and set guidelines for evaluation of the direction it finally takes. The Campaign, up to its launching on 2 April 1985, is documented and evaluated here. For the setting, there are the national newspapers of the time, in which the Drug Campaign was a major feature from December 1984 onwards.

Chapter 12   A national repertoire of action plans

Access to written material on drug education and drug abuse prevention programs is provided throughout this chapter, by source and phone number. For general sources, there are Alcohol and Drug Services and Health Promotion Services in every capital city, and nationally there is the library of the Alcohol and Drug Foundation, Australia in Canberra.

Some useful research articles on the general value of different types of intervention can be found in the literature. Examples are: Chappel et al., 'Substance abuse attitude changes in medical students' in *American journal of psychiatry*; Shattel and Carella, 'Macro-validation of training programs' in *Journal of drug education* (a model for training personnel on treatment of drug misuse); Northern Territory Department of Health's *The advertising of alcohol and tobacco products: the views and experience of the Northern Territory Drug and Alcohol Advisory Committee*; Frape and Tyler, *The North Coast Healthy Lifestyle Program 1979-1981*.

Chapter 13   The heart of the matter

In a sense the reading for this chapter is the previous dozen chapters of the book, since this last chapter is essentially a summary and review of what went before. If one could read only three books all told, we would suggest three prescribed for Chapter 1: those by Drew (editor), Nowlis and Weil. For those with an interest in where we are heading, there have been a series of commentators on our future, all of whom have something to offer: Toffler in *Previews and premises*, Roszak in *Where the wasteland ends*, Capra in *The turning point* and Ferguson in *The aquarian conspiracy*. None of these books are about drugs; all mention drugs in their proper, that is their cultural and historical, perspective.

Bibliography

Ackermann, A. (1983). Concerning bears, tigers and elephants: an exploration of health education in ACT schools, M.Ed. thesis, Canberra College of Advanced Education.

Addiction Research Foundation (1981). *Alcohol, public education and social policy.* Toronto.

Addiction Research Foundation (1981). *Task force on public education and social policy.* Toronto.

Auld, J. (1981). *Marihuana use and social control.* London: Academic Press.

Ausburn, L. (1979). *The pharmacist's role in improving patient compliance.* Sydney: Pharmaceutical Society of Australia, New South Wales Branch.

Australia. Commonwealth Department of Health (1984). *Annual report of the Director-General of Health 1983-84.* Canberra: Australian Government Publishing Service.

Australia. Department of Health. *Australian National Drug Information Service profiles.*

Australia. Department of Health (1984). *Alcohol in Australia: a summary of related statistics.* 3rd edn. Canberra: Australian Government Publishing Service.

Australia. Department of Health (1985). *Statistics on drug abuse in Australia.* Canberra: Australian Government Publishing Service.

Australia. Department of Health. Drugs of Dependence Branch (1984). *Abuse of volatile substances.* Information paper no. 4. Canberra: Australian Government Publishing Service.

Australia. Department of Health. Drugs of Dependence Branch (1984). *Cannabis: a review of some important national enquiries and significant research reports.* Canberra: Australian Government Publishing Service.

Australia. Department of Health. National Information Service on Drug Abuse (1982). Education for youth on the problems associated with drug use. *Technical information bulletin* 70: 16-20.

Australia. House of Representatives Standing Committee on Road Safety (1980). *Alcohol, drugs and road safety.* Canberra: Australian Government Publishing Service.

Australia. Royal Commission in to Intelligence and Security (1977-78). 4 reps. Canberra: Government Printer. (Commissioner: the Hon. Mr Justice R.M. Hope).

Australia. Senate Select Commission on Drug Trafficking and Drug Abuse (1971). *Report.* Canberra: Australian Government Publishing Service. (Chairman: Senator J.E. Marriott).

Australia. Senate Standing Committee on Social Welfare (1977). *Drug problems in Australia: an intoxicated society?* Canberra: Australian Government Publishing Service. (Chairman: Senator P. Baume).

Australian Bureau of Statistics. *Australian health survey 1977-78.* Canberra.

Australian Bureau of Statistics. *Australian health survey 1983: preliminary.* Canberra.

Australian Federal Police (1982). *Drug abuse in Australia, 1981.* Canberra: Government Printer.

Australian Foundation on Alcoholism and Drug Dependence (1981). National Workshop on Social Policies on Drugs, Canberra. Unpublished papers.

Australian Foundation on Alcoholism and Drug Dependence (1982). *Social policies on drugs: alcohol, cannabis, heroin.* Canberra.

Australian Royal Commission of Inquiry into Drugs (1980). Canberra: Australian Government Publishing Service. (Commissioner: the Hon. Mr Justice E.S. Williams).

Avery, G.S. (ed.) (1980). *Drug treatment.* 2nd edn. Sydney: Adis Press.

Balkin, G. (1983). The hotel of the future: patron care: threat or bonus to the industry. In: Carvolth, R. (ed.). *National Drug Institute: innovations.* Canberra: Australian Foundation on Alcoholism and Drug Dependence: 31-37.

Bandler, R. and Grinder, J. (1976). *The structure of magic: I and II.* Palo Alto, Ca: Science and Behaviour Books.

Barthes, R. (1975). *Mythologies.* London: Fontana Books.

Baume, P. (1977). See: Australia. Senate Standing Committee on Social Welfare.

Baume, P. (1984). *The buying of Australia.* South Melbourne: Alcohol and Drug Foundation, Victoria. (16th Leonard Ball Oration).

Bell, P. (1982). *Headlining drugs: an analysis of newspaper reports of drug-related issues in the N.S.W. press, 1980-81.* Surry Hills: New South Wales Drug and Alcohol Education and Information Centre.

Berne, E. (1978). *The games people play.* Harmondsworth: Penguin Books.

Beschner, G. and Thompson, P. (1981). *Women and drug abuse treatment: needs and services.* Rockville, Md: National Institute on Drug Abuse.

Bonnie, R.J. and Whitebread, C.H. (1970). Marihuana prohibition. *Virginia law review* 56: 971-1102.

Braithwaite, J. (1984). *Corporate crime in the pharmaceutical industry.* Melbourne: Routledge and Kegan Paul.

Briggs, G.G., Bondendorfer, T.W., Freeman, R.K. et al. (1983). *Drugs in pregnancy and lactation: a reference guide to fetal and neonatal risk.* Baltimore: Williams and Wilkins.

Broom (Darroch), D.H. (1978). Power and participation: the dynamics of medical encounters, Ph.D. thesis, Australian National University.

Brown, V.A. (1981). From sickness to health: an altered focus for health-care research. *Social science and medicine* 15A: 195-201.

Brown, V.A. (1985). Towards an epidemiology of health: a basis for planning community health programs. *Health policy* 4: 331-40.

Bulletin of narcotics (1983). Special issue on forfeiture of the proceeds of drug crimes. 35(2): Whole issue.

Burns, A. (1980). *Separation and divorce in Australia*. Melbourne: Nelson.

Cameron-Bandler, L. (1978). *They lived happily ever after*. Cupertino, Ca: Meta Publications.

Canada. Commission of Inquiry into the Non-medical Use of Drugs (1973). *Final report*. Ottawa: Information Canada. (Commissioner: G. Le Dain).

Capra, F. (1983). *The turning point: science, society and the rising culture*. New York: Bantam Books.

Carvolth, R. and Higgins, S. (1983). Hoteliers and health workers —strange bedfellows. In: Carvolth, R. (ed.). *National Drug Institute: innovations*. Canberra: Australian Foundation on Alcoholism and Drug Dependence: 63-66.

Castaneda, C. (1981). *The teachings of don Juan*. Harmondsworth: Penguin Books.

Centre for Education and Information on Drugs and Alcohol (1984). *An Australian handbook on drug use*. Canberra: Australian Government Publishing Service.

Chappel, J.N., Jordan, R.D., Treadway, B.J. and Miller, P.R. (1977). Substance abuse attitude changes in medical students. *American journal of psychiatry* 134: 379-84.

Connexions. Surry Hills: Centre for Education and Information on Drugs and Alcohol.

Cooper, J.R. et al. (eds) (1983). *Research on the treatment of narcotic addiction: state of the art*. Rockville, Md: National Institute on Drug Abuse.

Cox, T.C., Jacobs, M.R., Leblanc, A.E. et al. (1983). *Drugs and drug abuse*. Toronto: Addiction Research Foundation.

Darvall, L. (1984). Towards a comprehensive policy for prescription drug regulation. (Paper prepared for 11th World Congress of International Organisation of Consumers' Unions, Bangkok, 9-14 December 1984).

Davies, D.L. (ed.) (1977). *Epidemiological approach to the prevention of alcoholism symposium: the Ledermann curve*. London: Alcohol Education Centre.

Deveson. A. (1980). *Australians at risk*. Sydney: Cassell.

Dobinson, I. and Ward, P. (1985). *Drugs and crime: a survey of N.S.W. prison property offenders*. Sydney: N.S.W. Bureau of Crime Statistics and Research.

Douglas, M. (1970). *Purity and danger: an analysis of concepts of pollution and taboo*. London: Routledge and Kegan Paul.

Douglas, M. (1974). *Natural symbols*. Harmondsworth: Penguin Books.

Drew, L.R.H., Stoltz, P. and Barclay, W.A. (eds) (1981). *Man, drugs and society—current perspectives: proceedings of 1st Pan-Pacific Conference on Drugs and Alcohol*. Canberra: Australian Foundation on Alcoholism and Drug Dependence.

Drew, L.R.H. (1982). Death and drug use in Australia: 1969 to 1980. *Technical information bulletin* 69: 1-44.

Drew, L.R.H. (1983). Country profile: Australia. (Paper presented to WHO/WPRO Working Group on Prevention and Control of Drug Dependence, Manila, June/July 1983).

Drew, L.R.H. (1985). Alcohol and alcohol problems research in Australia. *British journal of addiction* (in press).

Dupont, R.L., Goldstein, A. and O'Donnell, J. (eds) (1979). *Handbook on drug abuse*. Rockville, Md: National Institute on Drug Abuse.

Edwards, G. and Arif, A. (eds) (1980). *Drug problems in the sociocultural context: a basis for policies and programme planning*. Geneva: World Health Organization.

Edwards, G., Awni, A. and Jaffe, J. (eds) (1983). *Drug use and misuse: cultural perspectives*. New York: St Martin's Press.

Einstein, S. (1983). Self-help drug misuse intervention: a schema. *International journal of the addictions* 18(4): 559-68.

Emery, F.E. and Emery, M. (1975). *A choice of futures: to enlighten or inform*. Canberra: Centre for Continuing Education, Australian National University.

Emery, F.E., Emery, M., Caldwell, G. and Crombie, A. (1975). *Futures we're in*. 1st rev. edn. Canberra: Centre for Continuing Education, Australian National University.

Erickson, P.G. (1980). *Cannabis criminals: the social effects of punishment on drug users*. Toronto: Addiction Research Foundation.

Erikson, E.H. (1968). *Identity: youth and crisis*. London: Faber and Faber.

Ferguson, M. (1981). *The aquarian conspiracy: personal and social transformation in the 1980's*. London: Granada.

Fisher, R. and Ury, W. (1983). *Getting to yes*. London: Hutchinson.

Foucault, M. (1978). *The history of sexuality*, vol. 1. Harmondsworth: Penguin Books.

Frape, G. and Tyler, C. (1984). *The North Coast Healthy Lifestyle Program 1979-1981*. Lismore: New South Wales Department of Health, North Coast Health Region.

Freed, A. (1976). *TA for teens*. Rolling Hills Estate, Ca: Jalmar Press.

Fry, D. and King, L. (School of Public Health and Tropical Medicine) (1985). *National Community Health Accreditation and Standards Project: final report*. Canberra: Australian Government Publishing Service.

Fuqua, P. (1978). *Drug abuse: investigation and control*. New York: McGraw Hill.

Garfield, E.F. and Gibbs, J. (1982). Fostering parent involvement for drug prevention. *Journal of drug education* 12 (2): 87-96.

Giddens, A. (1979). *Central problems in social theory: action, structure and contradiction in social analysis*. London: Macmillan.

Gilliland, K. and Bullock, W. (1983). Caffeine: a potential drug of abuse. *Advances in alcohol and substance abuse* 3(1/2): 53-74.

Glynn, T.J., Leukefeld, C.G. and Ludford, J.P. (eds) (1983). *Preventing adolescent drug abuse: intervention strategies*. Rockville, Md: National Institute on Drug Abuse.

Go ask Alice (1982). New York: Avon Books.

Goode, M. (1979). *Drugs and the law*. Adelaide: South Australian Royal Commission into the Non-medical Use of Drugs.

Goodman, L.S. and Gilman, A. (eds) (1980). *The pharmacological basis of therapeutics*. 6th edn. New York: Macmillan.

Goodstadt, M.S. (1980). Drug education—a turn on or a turn off? *Journal of drug education* 10(2): 89-99.

Gordon, T. (1974). *T.E.T.: teacher effectiveness training*. New York: Peter H. Wyden.

Gosselin, R.E., Smith, R.P. and Hodge, H.C. (1984). *Clinical toxicology of commercial products*. 5th edn. Baltimore: Williams and Wilkins.

Green, L. et al. (1980). *Health education planning: a diagnostic approach*. Palo Alto, Ca: Mayfield Publishing Company.

Gusfield, J. (1981). *The culture of public problems: drink-driving and the symbolic order*. Chicago: University of Chicago Press.

Habermas, J. (1971). *Knowledge and human interests*. Boston: Beacon Press.

Haynes, S. (1985). *Drugs in sport*. Canberra: Australian Sports Medicine Foundation.

Henderson, J. (1982). Substance use/abuse conceptualisation, etiology and treatment. *Journal of drug issues* 12(4): 317-32.

Hodgson, D. (1984). *The profits of crime and their recovery*. London: Heinemann.

Hope, R.M. (1977-78). See: *Australia. Royal Commission into Intelligence and Security*.

Huxley, A. (1932). *Brave new world*. New York: Harper and Row.

Huxley, A. (1965). *Brave new world revisited*. New York: Harper and Row.

Illich, I.D. (1965). *Medical nemesis*. London: Calder and Boyars.

Irwin, R.P. (1976). *Drug education programs and the adolescent in the drug phenomena problem*. Canberra: Australian National University.

Irwin, R.P. (1981). *Education and the use of alcohol and drugs*. South Melbourne: Victorian Foundation on Alcoholism and Drug Dependence. (13th Leonard Ball Oration).

Irwin, R.P. and Brown, V.A. (1981). Personal care and public good. *Australian family physician* 10: 536-41.

Irwin, R.P. (1983). Educational strategies in drug education: a focus for medical practitioners on the problems associated with alcohol and drug use. *Australian alcohol/drug review* 2(1): 10-13.

Irwin, R.P. (1984). Information, drugs, education and health. Canberra.

Jaffe, J. (ed.) (1983). *Drug use and misuse: cultural perspectives.* New York: St Martin's Press.

James, M. and Jongeward, D. (1971). *Born to win.* New York: Signet Books.

Kahn, T. (1969). *The structure of scientific revolutions.* Chicago: University of Chicago Press.

Kalant, O.J. (ed.) (1980). *Alcohol and drug problems in women* (Research advances in alcohol and drug problems, vol. 5). New York: Plenum Press.

Knowles, M. (1976). *The modern practice of adult education.* Chicago: Follett Publishing Company.

Kreek, M.J. and Stimmel, B. (eds) (1984). Dual addiction: pharmacological issues in the treatment of concomitant alcoholism and drug abuse. *Advances in alcohol and substance abuse* 3(4): Whole issue.

Krivanek, J.A. (1982). *Drug problems, people problems: causes, treatment and prevention.* Sydney: Allen and Unwin.

Lande, A. (1976). *Commentary on the convention on psychotropic substances.* New York: United Nations.

Lankton, S. (1980). *Practical magic.* Cupertino, Ca: Meta Publications.

Le Dain, G. (1973). See: Canada. Commission of Inquiry into the Non-medical Use of Drugs.

Ledermann, S. (1956). *Alcool-alcoolisme-alcoolisation: données scientifiques de caractère physiologique, economique et social.* Paris: Presses Universitaires de France.

Levi-Strauss, C. (1981). *Totem and taboo.* Harmondsworth: Penguin Books.

Lex, B.W. (1980). The recreational and social uses of dependency-producing drugs in diverse social and cultural contexts. *Journal of drug issues* 10(2): 159-63.

Logan, F. (ed.) (1979). *Cannabis: options for control.* Sunbury: Quartermaine.

Lusher, E.A. (1981). See: *New South Wales. Royal Commission into the New South Wales Police Force.*

MacDermott, K. (1981). Drug use surveys—no use to man or beast. In: Santamaria, J. (ed.). *Autumn school of studies on alcohol and drugs*. Melbourne: Department of Community Medicine, St Vincent's Hospital: 47-53.

McGregor, M., James, S., Gerrand, J. et al. (1982). *For love not money: a handbook for volunteers*. Blackburn, Vic.: Dove Communications.

MacIntyre, A. (1967). *A short history of ethics*. London: Routledge and Kegan Paul.

McLuhan, M. (1974). *Understanding media*. London: Abacus Books.

Marriott, J.E. (1971). See: Australia. Senate Select Commission on Drug Trafficking and Drug Abuse.

Martindale, W. (1982). *The extra pharmacopoeia*. 28th edn. London: Pharmaceutical Press.

Mead, M. (1978). *Culture and commitment: the new relationships between the generations in the 1970's*. New York: Columbia University Press.

Miller, G. and Agnew, N. (1974). The Ledermann model of alcohol consumption. *Quarterly journal of studies in alcohol* 35: 877-98.

Mills, C.W. (1959). *The sociological imagination*. New York: Oxford University Press.

Moffitt, A.R. (1974). See: *New South Wales. Royal Commission to Inquire in Respect of Certain Matters Relating to Allegations of Organised Crime in Clubs*.

Moser, J. (1980). *Prevention of alcohol-related problems*. Toronto: Alcoholism and Drug Dependence Research Foundation on behalf of World Health Organization.

Mugford, S. (1982). *An informal experiment in the price manipulation of low alcohol beer*. Sydney: New South Wales Drug and Alcohol Authority.

Mugford, S. (1983). Australian drinking patterns: a legacy for our children. In: Carvolth, R. (ed.). *National Drug Institute: innovations*. Canberra: Australian Foundation on Alcoholism and Drug Dependence: 21-26.

National Drug Education Program (1984). *Fourth report by 1983 assessment team of Drug Education Sub-Committee.* Canberra: Department of Health.

National Health and Medical Research Council (1978). *Report of the eighty-fourth session.* Canberra: Australian Government Publishing Service: 96-101.

National Health and Medical Research Council. Standing Committee on Health Promotion and Education. Sub-Committee on the Media and Health Promotion (1984). *The media and public health.* Canberra: NH&MRC.

National Heart Foundation (1985). *Risk-factor prevalence study, no. 2—1983.* Canberra: National Heart Foundation.

National Institute on Drug Abuse (1979). *Specialised therapeutic community programs for female addicts.* Rockville, Md.

National Working Party for the Drug Education Project (1982). *Guidelines for drug education.* Canberra: Curriculum Development Centre.

New South Wales. Report of the Royal Commission into Drug Trafficking (1979). Sydney: Government Printer. (Commissioner: the Hon. Mr Justice P.M. Woodward).

New South Wales. Royal Commission into the New South Wales Police Force (1981). Sydney: the Commission. (Commissioner: the Hon. Mr Justice E.A. Lusher).

New South Wales. Royal Commission to Inquire in Respect of Certain Matters Relating to Allegations of Organised Crime in Clubs (1974). Sydney: the Commission. (Commissioner: the Hon. Mr Justice A.R. Moffitt).

New South Wales Committee of Inquiry into the Legal Provision of Heroin and Other Possible Methods of Diminishing Crime Associated with the Supply and Use of Heroin (1981). *Report.* Sydney: Health Commission of New South Wales.

Noffs, T. (1985). *Life education centres: prevention as the ultimate answer to drug abuse.* Sydney: Wayside Foundation Publications.

Northern Territory Department of Health, Drug and Alcohol Bureau (1984). *The advertising of alcohol and tobacco products: the views and experience of the Northern Territory Drug and Alcohol Advisory Committee.* Darwin.

Nowlis, H. (1975). *Drugs demystified*. Paris: Unesco Press.

Nowlis, H. (1981). Prevention is not easy. In: Drew, L.R.H., Stoltz, P. and Barclay, W.A. (eds). *Man, drugs and society—current perspectives: proceedings of 1st Pan-Pacific Conference on Drugs and Alcohol.* Canberra: Australian Foundation on Alcoholism and Drug Dependence: 218-22.

O'Neill, K.A., Reilly, D.K. and Sinclair, R. (1984). Treatment of opioid dependence. *Australian alcohol/drug review* 4(1): 48-52.

Parlett, M. and Hamilton, D. (1972). *Evaluation as illumination.* Edinburgh: Centre for Research in the Educational Sciences, University of Edinburgh.

Pirsig, R. (1972). *Zen and the art of motorcycle maintenance.* New York: Corgi Books.

Polanyi, M. (1962). *Personal knowledge.* London: Routledge and Kegan Paul.

Polich, J.M., Ellickson, P.L., Reuter, P. and Kahan, J.P. (1984). *Strategies for controlling adolescent drug use.* Santa Monica, Ca: Rand.

Popper, K. (1973). *Objective knowledge.* London: Oxford University Press.

Rachin, R. (ed.) (1984). The orientation of sociology toward alcohol and society. *Journal of drug issues* 14(1): Whole issue.

Reynolds, I. and Rizzo, C. (1979). *Psychosocial problems of Sydney adults.* Sydney: Health Commission of New South Wales and Medicheck Referral Centre.

Ricketts, J. and Nanra, R.S. (1982). Analgesic abuse in perspective. *Australian alcohol/drug review* 1(1): 81-86.

Roger, K.M. (1982). Strategy for drug abuse prevention: the National Education Program. In: Wardlaw, G. (ed.). *Drug trade and drug use: proceedings of the conference presented by the Australian National University on drug trade and drug use, Canberra, Australia, October 22-24, 1980.* Canberra: Australian Foundation on Alcoholism and Drug Dependence for Australian National University: 29-37.

Room, R. (1983). Alcohol related problems: conceptual and methodological aspects. (Paper presented at 19th International Institute on the Prevention and Treatment of Alcoholism, Yugoslavia).

Room, R. (1984). An intoxicated society? Alcohol issues then and now in Australia. (Paper presented to International Group for Comparative Studies, Stockholm).

Roszak, T. (1973). *Where the wasteland ends: politics and transcendence in postindustrial society.* London: Faber and Faber.

Rowling, L. and Sparks, R.W. (1980). The role of the parent in the prevention of drug abuse. (Paper presented to 1st Pan-Pacific Conference on Drugs and Alcohol, Canberra).

Royal Commission of Inquiry into Drug Trafficking. Report (1983). Canberra: Australian Government Publishing Service. (Commissioner: the Hon. Mr Justice D.G. Stewart).

Rubin, V. (1975). *Cannabis and culture.* The Hague: Mouton.

Sackville, R. See: South Australian Royal Commission into the Non-medical Use of Drugs.

Santamaria, J. (ed.) (1979-84). *Autumn school of studies on alcohol and drugs.* Melbourne: Department of Community Medicine, St Vincent's Hospital.

Sargent, M. (1979). *Drinking and alcoholism in Australia: a power relations theory.* Melbourne: Longman Cheshire.

Sax, S. (1984). *A strife of interests: politics and policies in Australian health services.* Sydney: Allen and Unwin.

Schaps, E. et al. (1975-76). *Balancing head and heart: sensible ideas for the prevention of drug and alcohol abuse.* 3 vols. Lafayette, Ca: Prevention Materials Institute Press.

Schein, H. (1965). *Personal and organisational change.* New York: Wiley.

Schon, E. (1975). *Beyond the stable state.* Harmondsworth: Penguin Books.

Scott, D. (1981). *Don't mourn for me—organise: the social and political uses of voluntary organisations.* Sydney: Allen and Unwin.

Scriven, M. (1974). Pros and cons about goal-free evaluation. In: Popham, W.J. (ed.). *Evaluation in education: current applications.* Berkeley, Ca: McCutchan.

Shafer, R. See: United States. National Commission on Marihuana and Drug Abuse.

Sharpe, G. (1973). *The politics of non-violent action.* 3 vols. Boston: Extending Horizons Books.

Shattel, H.H. and Carella, S.C. (1976). Macro-validation of training programs. *Journal of drug education* 6: 193-200.

Simon, S.B., Howe, L.W. and Kirschenbaum, H. (1972). *Values clarification: a handbook of practical strategies for teachers and students.* New York: Hart.

Skog, O.-J. (1973). Less alcohol—fewer alcoholics? *Drinking and drug practices surveyor* 7: 7-13.

South Australian Royal Commission into the Non-medical Use of Drugs (1978). *Cannabis: a discussion paper.* Adelaide: the Commission. (Chairman: Prof. R. Sackville).

South Australian Royal Commission into the Non-medical Use of Drugs (1978). *The social control of drug use.* Adelaide: the Commission. (Chairman: Prof. R. Sackville).

South Australian Royal Commission into the Non-medical Use of Drugs (1979). *Final report.* Adelaide: the Commission. (Chairman: Prof. R. Sackville).

Stake, R.E. et al. (1975). *Evaluating the arts in education: a responsive approach.* Columbus, Ohio: Charles E. Merrill.

Stanton, M.D. (1979). Family treatment and drug problems. In: Dupont, R.L., Goldstein, A. and O'Donnell, J. (eds). *Handbook on drug abuse.* Rockville, Md: National Institute on Drug Abuse: 133-50.

State v. *Anonymous. Atlantic reporter* 2nd ser. 355: 729-42.

Stewart, D.G. (1983). See: *Royal Commission of Inquiry into Drug Trafficking. Report.*

Stimmel, B. (ed.) (1982). Evaluation of drug treatment programs. *Advances in alcohol and substance abuse* 2(1): Whole issue.

Stoltz, P. (1981). Present policies. (Paper prepared for National Workshop on Social Policies on Drugs, 7-9 April 1981, Canberra, sponsored by Social Policy Committee of Australian Foundation on Alcoholism and Drug Dependence).

Stufflebeam, D.L. (ed.) (1971). *Educational evaluation and decision-making.* Itasca, Ill.: F.E. Peacock.

Szasz, T.S. (1960). The myth of mental illness. *American psychologist* 15: 113-18.

Taylor, P. (1984). *Smoke ring: the politics of tobacco*. London: Bodley Head.

Taylor, R. (1980). *Medicine out of control*. Melbourne: Sun Books.

Time, F.M. and Ludford, J.P. (eds) (1984). *Drug abuse treatment evaluation: strategies, progress and prospects*. Rockville, Md: National Institute on Drug Abuse (NIDA research monograph no. 51: 13-28).

Titmuss, R.M. (1974). *Social policy: an introduction*. London: Allen and Unwin.

Toffler, A. (1972). *Future shock*. London: Pan Books.

Toffler, A. (1984). *Previews and premises*. London: Pan Books.

Toulmin, S. (1972). *Human understanding*, vol. 1. Oxford: Clarendon Press.

Trebach, A. (1983). Medicalised heroin and the British system. *US journal of drug and alcohol dependence* 7(5): 18-19.

Trelearen, G.K. and Thomas, J. (eds) (1981). *Prescription proprietaries guide*. 10th issue. Melbourne: Australian Pharmaceutical Publishing Company.

Trice, H.M. and Roman, P.M. (1978). *Spirits and demons at work: alcohol and other drugs on the job*. Ithaca, N.Y.: New York State School of Industrial and Labor Relations, Cornell University.

United Kingdom. Department of Health and Social Security (1982). *Treatment and rehabilitation: report of the Advisory Council on Misuse of Drugs*. London: HMSO.

United Nations. Commission on Narcotic Drugs (1984). *Report of the 8th session*. New York: United Nations.

United Nations Economic and Social Council (1982). *Review and implementation of the program of strategy and policies for drug control*. New York: United Nations.

United Nations Secretariat (1983). Preventive and treatment measures to reduce drug abuse: summary of responses to the survey of national programs. *Bulletin on narcotics* 35(3): 33-40.

United Nations Secretary General (1973). *Commentary on the single convention on narcotic drugs, 1961*. New York: United Nations.

United States. National Commission on Marihuana and Drug Abuse. 1st rep. (1972). *Marihuana, a signal of misunderstanding.* Washington, D.C.: the Commission. (Commissioner: R. Shafer).

United States. National Commission on Marihuana and Drug Abuse. 2nd rep. (1973). *Drug use in America: problem in perspective.* Washington, D.C.: the Commission. (Commissioner: R. Shafer).

Vessell, E.S. and Braude, M.C. (eds) (1976). Interactions of drugs of abuse. *Annals of the New York Academy of Science* 281: Whole issue.

Vuylsteek, K. (1979). *Health education: smoking, alcoholism, drugs.* Copenhagen: Euro reports and studies, World Health Organization.

Walker, R.B. (1984). *Under fire: a history of tobacco smoking in Australia.* Melbourne: Melbourne University Press.

Wardlaw, G. (1978). *Drug use and crime: an examination of drug users and associated persons and their influence on crime patterns in Australia.* Canberra: Australian Institute of Criminology.

Wardlaw, G. (ed.) (1982). *Drug trade and drug use: proceedings of the conference presented by the Australian National University on drug trade and drug use, Canberra, Australia, October 22-24, 1980.* Canberra: Australian Foundation on Alcoholism and Drug Dependence for Australian National University.

Weil, A. (1975). *The natural mind.* Harmondsworth: Penguin Books.

Wesson, D.R. and Smith, D.E. (1979). Treatment of the polydrug abuser. In: Dupont, R.L., Goldstein, A. and O'Donnell, J. (eds). *Handbook on drug abuse.* Rockville, Md: National Institute on Drug Abuse: 151-57.

Whyte, H.M. (1981). Psychological distress problems of community health, life style, drug use and health. Canberra: the author.

Williams, E.S. (1980). See: *Australian Royal Commission of Inquiry into Drugs.*

Williams, R.J. (1981). *The drug and alcohol court assessment program (DACAP).* Sydney: New South Wales Drug and Alcohol Authority.

Williams, R.J. and Bush, R. (1982). *Did the diversion of drug offenders fail in New South Wales?* Sydney: New South Wales Drug and Alcohol Authority.

Willis, E. (1983). *Medical dominance: the division of labour in Australian health care.* Sydney: Allen and Unwin.

Windschuttle, K. (1978). *Drugs and the press.* Adelaide: South Australian Royal Commission into the Non-medical Use of Drugs.

Woodward, P.M. (1979). See: *New South Wales. Report of the Royal Commission into Drug Trafficking.*

Working Party on the Management of Drug Using Women Who Are Pregnant and/or Who Have Young Children (1983). *Report.* Sydney: Health Commission of New South Wales.

World Health Organization (1982). Nomenclature and classification of drug and alcohol related problems: a shortened version of a WHO memorandum. *British journal of addiction* 77: 3-20.

Wyndham, D. (1981). My doctor gives me pills to put him out of my misery: women and psychotropic drugs. In: Drew, L.R.H. et al. (eds). *Man, drugs and society—current perspectives: proceedings of 1st Pan-Pacific Conference on Drugs and Alcohol.* Canberra: Australian Foundation on Alcoholism and Drug Dependence: 81-85.

Glossary

Action plan—outline of what has to be done, who has to do it, within what time frame and with what resources, and how it is to be evaluated.

Addiction—*see* **drug dependence.**

ADFA—Alcohol and Drug Foundation, Australia.

Alienation—lack of identification with family, job or society; at worst, lack of identification with self; emotional isolation.

Assessment—individual case analysis designed to provide the client with advice focusing on clear options for change. An adequate assessment distinguishes between problems derived from the origins of drug taking and problems derived from the consequences.

Community—a group of people who identify with the same set of symbols, rules and totems, and with each other.

Control—in standard use, legal methods aimed at suppressing, limiting or regulating drugs and users in general; planned actions directed towards creating or maintaining social order.

Culture—the mix of beliefs, practices and relationships which give the particular flavour we recognise as our own social world (not, as sometimes used, the art works of that social world).

DA:NA—Drugs in Australia: National Action. Title of a national drug workshop held in Canberra 24-27 February 1985 under the sponsorship of the Alcohol and Drug Foundation, Australia and the then Capital Territory Health Commission (now ACT Health Authority).

Drug—a chemical substance not normally present in the body which is ingested to meet a psychological, social or medical need.

Drug abuse—that use of a drug which is regarded by society as harmful to the individual or the society.

Drug dependence—a syndrome in which drug-taking behaviour assumes a much higher priority than other behaviours that once had higher value. Sensory neurone adaptation (alias addiction) is a type of dependence in which physical withdrawal symptoms develop once drug taking has stopped.

Education—the process of learning something new: can take place at any age in any setting, not only in formal settings.

Hard drugs—the long-standing illegal drugs, such as narcotics, which link the user to the criminal and antisocial elements of society.

Intervention—a broadly encompassing term for any action directed to bringing about change.

Legalisation—legal steps to reduce the sanctions applied to the use and availability of drugs. Removal of sanctions does not necessarily occur *in toto*; it may be partial or gradual.

Means—the mechanisms by which we reach a stated or unstated goal; often confused with the *ends,* that is, the goal itself.

Media—shorthand for mass media, the avenues used for transmitting public messages: newspapers, pamphlets, television, videotapes and radio are each a medium of mass communication.

NCADA—National Campaign Against Drug Abuse

Peer group—members of a group who regard each other as equals in some respect: image, status, sporting prowess, drug use or educational level.

Policy—established principles which govern action directed towards stated ends.

Possession—a legal term which refers to custody of a proscribed substance (with the implication of personal use).

Prevention—anticipatory steps taken to avoid consequences perceived as harmful.

Promotion—in the case of health promotion, any educational, organisational, economic or political intervention designed to improve health.

Social context—a perspective on drug use which varies depending on the standpoint of the groups or individuals involved.

Society—the institutions, rules, habits, norms and roles by which people construct their social environment.

Strategy—guidelines for the actions required to give effect to policy.

Supply—the physical availability of a drug and the legal limits on it. Controls on supply can be distinguished from controls on demand, which are considered to be measures taken to influence people's choice with regard to drug use.

Taboo—objects or behaviours which are so thoroughly forbidden that they are never considered or mentioned (as faeces or incest).

Totem—symbol of a rule that must be respected because it reflects deeply held beliefs (as in American Indians' pole carvings of sacred figures, or the Australian dream home).

Traffic—entrepreneurial activity within the drug market place.

Treatment—a body of practices whose principal characteristic is the goal of changing the individual's behaviour in a definably desirable way.

Index

aborigines, 33, 43, 197, 211, 220-221, 223, 239
  analgesic use, 82
  other drug use, 33
  pitcheri use, 23
ACT needs, 40, 185-187
action, 13, 89-90, 163-255
Addiction Research Foundation of Ontario, 231
ADFA *see* Alcohol and Drug Foundation, Australia
administration of drugs, 60
Adolescent Medical Unit, Camperdown, 224, 228
Advertising, 39, 110-111, 150-151, 251
  alcohol, 200, 246
  tobacco, 200-201
aesthetic standards, 171, 183, 193
AIDS, 46
Al-Anon Family Groups, 245
Alateen, 244
Alcohol: Its Science and Sociology, 229
alcohol abuse, 42, 192
Alcohol and Drug Authority, WA, 238, 239, 240, 242, 253
Alcohol and Drug Dependence Service, Qld, 253
Alcohol and Drug Dependency Board, Tas, 253
Alcohol and Drug Foundation, Australia, 153, 216, 248, 252
Alcohol and Drug Programs Unit, Qld, 221, 236, 240
Alcohol and Drug Service, ACT, 225, 252

alcohol drinking, 73-74, 260
  price and availability, 112, 250
Alcohol, Drug and Forensic Branch, Vic, 237, 242, 253
'Alcohol Education' (program), 231
alcoholic beverage industry, 30
Alcoholics Anonymous, 121, 244
'All about me' (program), 230
amphetamines, 65
AMSAD, 237, 249
analgesics, 38, 81-82
apprentices, 225
attitudes, 23, 79
  of doctors, 52
Australian Advertising Industry Council, 252
Australian Associated Brewers, 248
Australian Bureau of Criminal Intelligence, 213
Australian Alcohol/Drug Review (journal), 237
Australian Broadcasting Tribunal, 246
Australian Health Surveys, 80-81
Australian Institute of Criminology, 249
Australian Medical Society on Alcohol and Drug Related Problems, 237, 249
Australian Sports Medicine Federation, 146, 243

barbiturates, 68, 84, 192
Baume, Peter, 13, 41-43, 51
Belconnen Care Education, 225

INDEX 301

Bell, Philip, 191
benzodiazepines, 80
Best of friends (video), 240
Blewett, Neal, 34-36, 168
blood alcohol level, 200, 251
Body Owners' Program, 230
BUGA-UP, 158, 223
BYO (video), 240

CADAP *see* Community Approach to Drug Abuse Prevention
caffeine, 62, 64, 76, 194
Campbell, Elizabeth, 226
cannabis, 17, 62, 70
　criminal charges, 113
　decriminalisation, 108, 177, 184, 186
　expunging of criminal record for possession of, 184, 204
　legalisation, 97-100, 107-109
　seizures, 114
　use, 70, 85, 188, 194
case studies, 124-125
CASPAR, 233
Centre for Education and Information on Drugs and Alcohol, 191, 230
CHASP, 148
civil liberties, 53, 100, 104
coastal surveillance, 102, 213
cocaine, 66, 113
coercion, 106-107, 124
Cole, Judy, 222
Community Approach to Drug Abuse Prevention, 147, 221
community education, 193, 204, 218-223
Community Health Education Campaign, 219
community intervention, 51, 142-144, 154, 182
community workshops, 184-185, 187-188
confiscation of assets, 199, 212
Connexions (newletter), 188
consumer organisations, 156-157
control, 15-17, 57, 97-115
Convention on Psychotropic Substances, 99
corrective services, 182, 203
corruption, 200
crime, 191, 200, 250
criminal charges, 113

Crowley, Rosemary, 38-39
CSIRO Division of Human Nutrition, 230
curriculum development, 130
customs, 101, 214

DACAP, 251
DA:NA *see* Drugs in Australia: National Action
data collection, 182, 202
Datura, 23, 62, 63
'Decision-making Skills about Legal and Illegal Drugs', 231
Department of Education, Northern Territory, 225
dependence, 30-31, 61
depressants, 59, 66-69
detoxification, 120-121, 186, 187
diversion of offenders, 106, 177, 186, 199
dosage, 60
Drew, Les, 13, 112
drink drivers, 186
drink driving education, 222, 226-227, 246
driving, 214
Drug and Alcohol Authority, NSW, 222, 225, 226, 252
Drug and Alcohol Bureau, NT, 229, 253
Drug and Alcohol Court Assessment Program, 251
Drug and Alcohol Services Council, SA, 219, 225, 237, 241, 253
'Drug summit' (Special Premiers' Conference, 2 April, 1985), 45, 168, 210-214
drug trafficking, 213
drug use, 27
　effects, 59-71
　statistics, 42, 72-86
　surveys, 202
　see also mortality; names of specific drugs
drugs, definition, 59
Drugs in Australia: National Action, 15-16, 43, 140, 176-182, 194
　evaluation, 183-184
　participants, 205-207
　recommendations, 196-204
　workshop design, 207-209
drugs in sport, 82, 92, 243
Drugs in the Family (program), 245

education, 15, 17, 130-140, 182, 188, 198-199, 211-212
see also community education; training of addictions workers
effectiveness training, 137
Emery, Fred, 157
Enmore High School, 228
Ethanol, 66
ethical goals, 171, 183, 192
ethnic drug users, 33
evaluation, 172-174
of treatment services, 125-126

facts, definition, 91
families, 33, 143, 186, 198
Family Interaction Program, 234
Family Living, 245
Fmily Medicine Program, 239
fear, 30
FMECH, 150
foetus, drug effects, 62, 171
forfeiture of assets, 104
funding, 211
Free to Choose (program), 241

general practitioners, 52, 117, 185
glue sniffing, 58, 242
Hackett, Earle, 97, 149, 270-272
Health Education News and Views (newsletter), 242
Health Education Unit, Sydney Institute of Education, 236
Health Promotion Branch, ACT Health Authority, 223, 229, 241
'Here's Looking at You, Two', 233
heroin, 98, 124, 186, 192
legalisation, 35, 100, 177, 182, 261-262
seizure, 114
treatment, 35, 203, 212
See also methadone
Hewitson, M, 229
homeless, 32
holistic models, 92-96, 159-162
'Hooked on Health' Week, 228
hospital admissions, drug related, 73
hotels, 152

identity cards, 252
Institute for the Study of Drug Dependence, 231
international treaties, 99

Jaffe, J, 28

Karralika, 186
Kelly, Ros, 40-41

Latrobe Valley Community Smoking Control Project, 249
law enforcement, 213, 250-252
Ledermann, S, 53
legal drugs *see* alcohol, tobacco, therapeutic drugs, analgesics etc.
legalisation, 97-98, 100-101
see also under names of specific drugs
legislation, 212-213
Levi-Strauss, C, 6
licensing laws, 200, 250, 252
licit vs illicit drugs, 35, 38, 41, 53, 106, 182, 189, 258
'Life. Be in it' campaign, 114
Life Education Centre, 226
lifestyle, 223
Lions/ADFA Foundation, 219
Lions Clubs, 219
longitudinal studies, 202
low alcohol beer, 15
LSD, 62, 63, 168

Mackay inquest, 191
marihuana *see* cannabis
McLuhan, M, 169
Mead, Margaret, 141
media, 39, 42-43, 103, 147-149, 152, 182, 185, 189-191
campaigns, 201-202, 245-247
Medical Education Project, 238
metabolism, 60
methadone, 36, 97, 122-123, 138, 177, 182, 186, 190, 204, 212
Ministerial Council on Drug Strategy, 211
modelling, 138, 258
moral values, 184
moral/legal approach, 28, 54
mortality, 42, 75, 82, 84

narcotics, 69, 82, 84
criminal charges, 113
see also heroin
Narcotics Anonymous, 121, 244
narcotics users, 32

National Alcohol and Drug Dependence Industry Program, 153, 221
National Campaign Against Drug Abuse 12, 41, 43, 140, 175-195, 214
submissions, 189
National Drug Education Program, 40, 51, 133-134, 186, 224
National Health and Medical Research Council, 248
national policy, 45-58, 175-176
National Safety Council, 222
Natural Helpers Program, 232
negotiation skills, 158
Neurolinguistics, 137
nicotine, 64, 192
Noffs, Ted, 226
North Coast Healthy Lifestyle Program, 149, 217, 222
Nowlis, Helen, 13
NSW Bureau of Crime Statistics and Research, 249
Nurses Education Project, 238, 241

Odyssey House, 158, 244
Operation Noah, 191
Operation Oldies, 222
opium production, 99

painkillers *see* analgesics
Pallister House, 243, 247
paracetamol, 62
parenting, 145
Patron Care Program, 152, 219
PCP, 62, 63
Peer Support Foundation, 226
peer support programs, 188
petrol sniffing, 229, 242
Pharmacy Guild of Australia, 219
Phoebe House, 171, 173, 245
pitcheri, 23
police powers, 104
policy, 13, 45, 181, 196-197
control as policy, 115
education as policy, 139
prevention as policy, 160
treatment as policy, 129
political party policy, 48-50
politicians, 34
possession, 105-106
Pregnant Pause Campaign, 135, 220

prescriptions, 80, 82, 250
prevention of drug problems, 139, 142, 197, 215-255
price, 250
prisons, prisoners, 106, 203
programs, 219-253
definition, 217
projects definition, 217-218
psychedelic drugs, 59, 63
psycho-social approach, 56
public health approach, 28, 56, 116-117

'Quit. For Life' campaign, 244, 247

random breath testing, 110, 200, 250
registers of drug users, 182, 202
registration of addicts, 190
rehabilitation, 187, 203-204, 244
of offenders, 203
research, 200, 202, 212, 247-249
resources, 239-243
Richmond Fellowship, 155
Richmond, Robyn, 239
risk taking, 86
Road Traffic Authority, Vic, 227
Room, Robin, 13, 29
Royal Commissions, 8-11, 43, 51, 53, 133

School of Community Medicine, UNSW, 239
Search conferences, 157-158
self help groups, 144, 155-158
self regulation, 251-252
sentencing, 186, 251
services, definition, 218
SICH, 148
side effects, 62
Single Convention on Narcotic Drugs, 99
smoking, 76-77, 110, 224, 227, 239
Smoking and Health Project, WA, 227
Smoking Cessation Program, 239
Smoking Education Project, Qld, 228
snakes and ladders, 264-267
social change, 15-17, 141-163
social context, 14, 21-43, 165, 181
social rules, 171, 183
socio-cultural approach, 29, 56

Solvent Abuse Education Program, 242
Special Premiers' Conference *see* 'Drug summit'
sponsorship
  sports, 111, 201, 246
sport, 146 *see also* drugs in sport; sponsorship
STARR Project, 234
stimulants, 59, 65-66
strategy, 13, 87-96, 171, 181
Street Leaders Camp, 229
Student Council Stop Smoking Project, 229
students, 223-234
  drug use, 79
Substance Abuse Monthly (newsletter), 242
Sumner Tobacco and Alcohol Risk Reduction Project, 234
supply, 101
surveys, 202

taxation, 200, 250
telephone counselling, 212
therapeutic communities, 121
therapeutic drugs, 77-81 *see also* analgesics, depressants, stimulants, tranquillisers
'Think well' program, 230
Tic-tac totem, 21
tobacco industry, 30, 110
tolerance, 61
Toronto Board of Education, 231
totems and taboos, 3, 6-7, 21-23, 72, 97, 117-118, 139, 161-162, 194, 256-259
training of addictions workers, 133, 149-150, 185, 199, 234-239

trafficking, 102-104, 210, 213
tranquillisers, 5, 67, 81, 192, 261
transactional analysis 137
treatment 15-17, 38-39, 116-129, 187, 188, 203-204, 212
  agencies, 110
  client/treatment matching, 118
  drug free goal, 118, 125
  evaluation, 123-124
  see also subheading: treatment under specific drug names
trust, 30

underage drinking, 252
unemployed, 32

values, 91-93, 193
values clarification, 136-137
vested interests, 29
volatile substance abuse, 71, 85, 110
  see also glue sniffing
voluntary agencies, 154-155, 237

Webster, Ian W, 239
Westchester County Student Assistance Program, 232
'Why smoke' (program), 217, 224-225
Whyte, Malcolm, 28
Woma Committee, 223
women, 187, 211
workplace, 153
World Health Organisation, 215
Wran, Neville, 188

youth, 72, 175, 211, 252
Youth Life Project, 224